Early Diagnosis
and Therapy
in Cerebral Palsy

PEDIATRIC HABILITATION

series editor ALFRED L. SCHERZER

Cornell University Medical Center
New York, New York

vol. 1   **Prevention of Mental Retardation and Other Developmental Disabilities,**
         edited by Michael K. McCormack

vol. 2   **Developmental Disabilities: Management through Diet and Medication,**
         Eric Denhoff and Steven A. Feldman

vol. 3   Early Diagnosis and Therapy in Cerebral Palsy: A Primer on Infant
         Developmental Problems, Alfred L. Scherzer and Ingrid Tscharnuter

Additional Volumes in Preparation

Early Diagnosis and Therapy in Cerebral Palsy

A Primer on Infant Developmental Problems

ALFRED L. SCHERZER
INGRID TSCHARNUTER

MARCEL DEKKER, INC.   New York and Basel

Library of Congress Cataloging in Publication Data

Scherzer, Alfred L.
    Early diagnosis and therapy in cerebral palsy.

    (Pediatric habilitation; v. 3)
    Includes indexes.
    1. Cerebral palsied children. I. Tscharnuter,
Ingrid, [date]. II. Title. III. Series.
[DNLM: 1. Cerebral palsy—Diagnosis. 2. Cerebral
palsy—Therapy. W1 PE167K v. 3 / WS 342 S326e]
RJ496.C4S344 1982   618.92'836   82-13043
ISBN 0-8247-1828-3

MARCEL DEKKER, INC.
270 Madison Avenue, New York, New York 10016

Current printing (last digit):
10 9 8 7 6

PRINTED IN THE UNITED STATES OF AMERICA

*To the many children and their families
from whom we have learned so much,
and who have enabled us to share with others*

Preface

Until relatively recent years, cerebral palsy was primarily of professional interest to a limited number of specialists dealing with specific aspects of treatment, such as orthopedics and neurology. Indeed, these are the specialties which initially shaped its definition and scope, dating from the days of Little and Freud. Children came to attention late, when significant limitations in development and milestones were noted, or severe orthopedic deficits were apparent. Intervention was frequently concerned with static neurologic assessment, and treatment often exclusively focused upon orthopedic surgery or a form of limited individual muscle therapy. The approach was to deal with the specific functional deficits as they appeared.

A much broader concept has subsequently emerged with the awareness that cerebral palsy represents a major multidisciplinary developmental disorder in which timely intervention by a variety of specialties is essential, and a coordinated, directed approach is required. In addition, traditional therapy involving individual muscle training has given way—mostly through clinical work with cerebral palsy—to a more comprehensive and dynamic approach of movement education which emphasizes the sensorimotor duality and is therefore conducive to learning new motor skills. Clinical experience with cerebral palsy has also promoted an expansion in the understanding of sensorimotor development. Today, abnormal motor behavior typically associated with cerebral palsy is seen as the outcome of a long process of postural compensations to underlying deficits, such as abnormal postural tonus or poor integration of postural reflexes. While early and primary postural compensations consist of more subtle deviations from the norm, motor skills building on these deviant patterns become more and more abnormal.

Newer knowledge concerning infant development and recognition of early common findings among infants with nonprogressive central nervous system deficits has now placed cerebral palsy within the spectrum of major developmental disabilities. In fact, its early identification and management presently serve as a model for other types of multiply handicapping conditions.

Recent perinatal management and neonatal intensive care technologies have further influenced the outlook for the child with potential disability. Children are now surviving who until recently had an abysmal prognosis. Evidence indicates a reduction, as well, in degree of disability, although an increase in severity is suggested especially among those high-risk and low-birth-weight infants who formerly did not survive. It seems likely that chronic developmental disorders in children are destined to be a major and increasing concern for pediatrics of the future.

It is in this setting that the concepts of early diagnosis and intervention have taken root and a sizable literature has emerged. Current data are clinically supportive of early intervention and the notion is intuitively appealing on the basis of developmental theory. An explosive interest has been generated in this field, yet there is a paucity of sources available for comprehensive reference and documentation.

The present text attempts to fill this gap by putting into perspective the evolution of cerebral palsy from a narrow focus as an orthopedic disability to a broadly conceived developmental disorder. The emphasis is on the process of developmental diagnosis, and current clinical approaches to evaluation, management, and treatment are detailed. The need for continuous, systematic, and standardized re-evaluation is stressed. Suggestions are made for developing research methods which will ultimately lead to establishing the effectiveness of any given treatment approach.

It is hoped that the text will provide a useful guide for those who deal with a wide variety of developmental disabilities in young children. Considerable emphasis is placed on identifying early patterns of postural maladjustments so that they can be corrected as far as possible before leading to more severe abnormalities. Its focus is to provide a more uniform and standardized approach to diagnosis and treatment. Only in this way will it be possible to objectively evaluate and guide individual therapy activities. Ultimately, this will greatly aid in the much needed quest for research methodologies and firm data concerning the early intervention process.

Alfred L. Scherzer
Ingrid Tscharnuter

Contents

Preface   v

1. Definition of Cerebral Palsy and Scope of the Problem   1

2. Developmental Evaluation and Differential Diagnosis   21

3. Planning for the Abnormally Developing Child   53

4. Normal and Abnormal Sensorimotor Development   *73*

5. Neurodevelopmental Assessment of Infants: Concepts   123

6. Neurodevelopmental Assessment of Infants: Procedures   145

7. Home Management   163

8. Treatment   205

9. Assessment of the Management-Treatment Program   257

Author Index   279

Subject Index   285

Early Diagnosis and Therapy in Cerebral Palsy

1
Definition of Cerebral Palsy and Scope of the Problem

CEREBRAL PALSY IN HISTORICAL PERSPECTIVE

While the physician Cazauvielh was the first to study cerebral paralysis scientifically [1], an orthopedic surgeon had the earliest professional interest in cerebral palsy and his influence has continued to help shape the basis for treatment. Delpech was concerned with the deformities resulting from poliomyelitis and was the first to describe the tendo Achillis lengthening for equinus [2]. The procedure caught the interest of John Little, an English orthopedist who himself had contracted polio that left a residual equinus deformity (Fig. 1). Little consulted Delpech about the operation but was discouraged because of possible complicating infection. He subsequently went to Germany, where the procedure was also being developed, and underwent a successful operation.

Little was impressed with the tendo Achillis lengthening and became adept at the procedure upon his return to England. He also became increasingly interested in correction of various deformities in children [3]. Among these conditions he began to recognize many associated with paralysis and particularly with generalized spasticity [4]. His definitive work in 1861 drew upon twenty years' experience and documented correlations between abnormality

Figure 1 W. John Little, English orthopedist whose studies of cerebral palsy formed the basis of modern treatment.

of pregnancy, labor, delivery, and subsequent developmental deficit [5]. Little reasoned that spasticity and deformity were due to cerebral hemorrhage secondary to trauma of the birth process (Fig. 2). Little's disease had thus become established.

Interest in the condition spread to other medical disciplines. Gowers was among the earliest physicians to support Little's view [6]. Osler showed the neuroanatomical correlation of structural brain pathology and spastic paralysis [7].

Contraction of adductors and flexors of lower extremities. Left hand weak. Both hands awkward. More paralytic than spastic. Born with navel-string around neck. Asphyxia neonatorum one hour. See Case XLIII.

Figure 2 Little related paralysis and spasticity in children to birth trauma (from Ref. 5).

Figure 3 Sigmund Freud studied nonprogressive neurological deficits and prematurity in children.

Freud, as a neurologist concerned with children, became greatly interested in the relationship of nonprogressive neurological deficits and prematurity [8]. He placed greater emphasis on intrauterine developmental abnormality and less on trauma than had Little (Fig. 3).

The interest in identification and etiology of spastic conditions initiated in the latter part of the nineteenth century maintained only limited momentum early into the twentieth century. Specific approaches to treatment were also slow in developing and had relatively little impact. Physical therapy made a start in the United States through the work of Jennie Colby at Children's Hospital in Boston [9]. She was a gymnast with interest in massage and developed remedial exercises for a variety of paralytic conditions. The work was purely empirical and was incorporated into the newly emerging neurology clinic established by Crothers. Here the new dimensions of psychological aspects and mental health were added by Elizabeth Lord [10].

Orthopedic surgery to correct specific deformity gained further popularity through the work of Stoffel. He perfected neurectomy as a specific procedure for managing contractures [11]. Surgery was viewed enthusiastically because of the easily measurable immediate and selected improvement. However, initial surgical benefit was often followed by disappointing long-term results.

As the psychological, developmental, neurological, and surgical considerations became more apparent, a broader approach was needed. The impetus started with Crothers and the interdisciplinary model in Boston. This was greatly expanded by Winthrop Phelps, an orthopedist who became devoted to the needs of handicapped children, and who ultimately established a comprehensive community rehabilitation center in Maryland [12]. Phelps demonstrated the multispecialty approach in the period before World War II, when there was relatively little interst within the medical field.

The years immediately after the war brought together extensive experience with rehabilitation medicine and rapid maturation in a variety of medical specialties. A renewed interest in the handicapped child became apparent in a number of professional groups. Community demand had begun to stir. The National Society for Crippled Children and Adults (Easter Seal Society) set up a Cerebral Palsy Division in 1946 with a National Advisory Medical Council. This group of professionals quickly recognized the need for a forum for interdisciplinary information and exchange of ideas.

It was in this setting that the American Academy for Cerebral Palsy (AACP) was born in Chicago in 1947 [13]. Conceived as a multispecialty professional organization to stimulate research and training in the field of the handicapped child, the AACP joined together the major medical disciplines with related therapy, educational, and psychological services. The founders, all of whom were in the original Easter Seal Group, had become convinced that only a combined effort could hope to have a measurable impact (Fig. 4).

Figure 4 The founders of the American Academy for Cerebral Palsy, 1947.
Standing (left to right): Dr. George Deaver (physiatrist), Dr. Earl Carlson
(internist), Dr. Meyer Perlstein (pediatrician). Seated (left to right): Dr.
Dr. Bronson Crothers (neurologist), Dr. Winthrop Phelps (orthopedist),
Dr. Temple Fay (neurophysiologist).

They included Phelps, who was the first president, Temple Fay (neurophysiologist), Bronson Crothers (neurologist), Meyer Perlstein pediatrician),
George Deaver (physiatrist), and Earl Carlson (internist). What started as a
small forum for discussion and interprofessional education was the beginning
of a midcentury resurgence of interest and effort on behalf of the handicapped child [14].

Demand for local services and facilities occurred simultaneously. A local
cerebral palsy committee was established in New York in *1948* [15]. It
sponsored local hospital diagnostic services and provided treatment and educational programs based largely on the model developed in Maryland by
Phelps in the 1930s. A New York State and finally a national United Cerebral Palsy Association followed with the subsequent development of more
than 300 local chapters throughout the United States [16].

Of necessity, the emphasis of these programs was on diagnosis and treatment of the child with established deficits: frequently severe deformity of a long-standing nature. Children were being seen with deformity comparable to Little's experience of a century before. The difference lay in an approach much broader than orthopedics alone. In addition to the medical specialties, psychological services, and therapies, serious effort was being made to provide appropriate special education, needed supportive social service, and family mental health programs. As services developed and identification of the already handicapped became more efficient, there has been an increasing trend from a rehabilitative to a "habilitative" approach. This aims to employ whatever means necessary to bring a child to a level of maximum potential in all areas of development, and particularly to ensure functional independence as an individual.

Technological developments in perinatal care from the late 1960s to the present have added further impetus to this concept. Improvement in obstetrical management of the high-risk mother has combined with a system of intensive neonatal care to reduce mortality significantly and selectively lower morbidity from neurological and developmental deficit [17]. More "at-risk" infants are living and emergence of more effective methods of identification of early neurological abnormality increasingly is accompanying this trend. Contributions from developmental psychology and neurology, and experience of transdisciplinary methods with very young children have been particularly influential [18].

A parallel and logical outcome is early intervention treatment. While still imperfect in many respects, the present system of care has generally "caught up" with the late case of untreated and multiple deficit. In this respect, the goals of the 1950s to treat those with existing definitive handicaps are being met. As is seen in management of many medical conditions, the initial emphasis and interest lies with the most obvious and severe forms of the condition. As these become treated and greater understanding of cause is approached, emphasis is placed on more subtle forms and, finally, early diagnosis and treatment. So it is with cerebral palsy as we enter the 1980s. The data on the effect of early intervention are just emerging but clearly are encouraging [19].

In a period of slightly more than 100 years there has been a virtual revolution in concept and thought concerning cerebral palsy. Conceived initially as an orthopedic deficit with a neurological basis, it has come to be recognized as a multihandicapping condition requiring many specialties and services. But more than this, it is seen as a major disorder in development—a disability which emerges as the child grows—requiring early identification and management. Thus the orthopedic disease has become the prototype of the developmental disability and has helped open up a better understanding of the dynamics of developmental problems in children.

Recognition of this broader concept was given in 1977 when the AACP officially became the American Academy for Cerebral Palsy and Developmental Medicine (AACPDM) [20]. Little's early concern for the deformed child has at last merged with the broad area of the developmentally disabled.

TOWARD A DEFINITION OF CEREBRAL PALSY

Much confusion continues to exist concerning the term cerebral palsy and its accepted meaning. Cerebral palsy refers to a *nonprogressive* central nervous system deficit. The lesion may be in a single or multiple locations of the brain, resulting in definite motor and possibly sensory abnormality. It occurs as a result of inutero factors, events at the time of labor and delivery (congenital cerebral palsy), or a variety of factors in the early developing years (acquired cerebral palsy). The former is estimated to account for 85 percent and the latter 15 percent of cases [21].

The term cerebral palsy was first used by Burgess in 1888 [22]. This was closely followed in the English literature by Osler [7], Sachs and Peterson [23], in France by Brissaud [24], and among the infuential Germans by Rosenberg [25], and Freud [26]. Phelps was the major popularizer in the United States. In conjunction with Phelps' work in developing a comprehensive treatment program, cerebral palsy came to be known as the major nonprogressive motor deficit in children [27]. The AACPDM and the United Cerebral Palsy Associations have both reinforced the developmental aspects of the definition [28].

In addition to the motor deficit, other associated handicaps are frequently present. These include abnormalities of vision (twenty-five percent) [29], hearing and speech (greater than fifty percent) [30], seizure disorders (one-third) [31], mental retardation (fifty to seventy-five percent depending on motor severity) [32], learning disabilities among the vast majority, and frequent social, emotional, and interfamily problems. In every sense, therefore, the term conveys the concept of a multiply handicapping condition.

Confusion of terms and overlapping with other nonprogressive central nervous system (CNS) disorders may be present. Cerebral palsy is a static *motor* deficit with associated handicaps. The primary *motor* nature of the condition provides a clear separation from mental retardation syndromes, organic brain deficits, autism, or emotional disorders.

CLASSIFICATION OF CEREBRAL PALSY MOTOR TYPES

The motor pattern type of cerebral palsy may take several forms. The spastic variety is most common and indicates a fixed lesion in the motor portion of the cerebral cortex. Athetosis or dystonia reflects involvement in the basal

Table 1 Distribution of Cerebral Palsy Types

Location	Description
Monoplegia	One extremity
Hemiplegia	Upper and lower extremity on one side
Paraplegia	Both lowers
Quadriplegia	Equal involvement of uppers and lowers
Diplegia	Quadriplegia with mild upper involvement

ganglia. Frequently it involves intermittent tension of trunk or extremities and a variety of uninhibited movement patterns—sometimes a basis for confusion in classification. Ataxia relates to a cerebellar lesion. Mixed types are also common. These may include combinations of spasticity with athetosis or ataxia. Rigidity suggests a severe decerebrate lesion.

The clinical neurological lesion has variable distribution. Table 1 indicates definitions in common use.

Severity must also be considered as a basis for description and guide for prognosis and treatment. A descriptive statement should at least indicate that the involvement is mild, moderate, or severe.

Type, distribution, and severity are essential aspects of the cerebral palsy diagnosis. They give meaning and direction to treatment and management of the patient, and provide a more uniform understanding of the problem than simply referring to a static motor encephalopathy.

Classification and uniformity of diagnostic description has always been controversial. Rosenberg was the first to tackle the problem [25]. He included these categories: generalized rigidity, paraplegic rigidity, bilateral spastic hemiplegia, bilateral athetosis, chorioform diplegia, and atypical forms.

Freud [26] made a slight refinement. He gave more recognition to athetosis. Categories included spastic hemiplegia, generalized rigidity, paraplegic rigidity, paraplegic paralysis, double hemiplegia, generalized chorea, and bilateral athetosis.

These were the only classifications available until the mid-twentieth century and were largely the basis for understanding and describing the lesions up to that time. The modern era in classification dates from 1950 and the work of Fay [33]. He greatly elaborated on various clinical aspects of the movement disorder, perhaps encumbering the system beyond practical use:

Spastic paralysis—cerebral Nonspastic paralysis; atonic type

Athetosis—midbrain Deafness; tension; nontension; hemiplegia; tremor; cerebral release; emotional release; head, neck, arm; shudder-type; rotary-type; dystonia type; flail-type

Tremors and rigidities—basal ganglia Parkinsonism types; decerebrate types

Ataxia cerebellar; kinesthetic

High spinal spastic—medulla

Mixed—difuse

Phelps greatly refined these categories into a simpler and more practical clinical scheme [34]. He included the following: flaccid paralysis, spasticity, rigidity, tremor, athetosis, and ataxia. This system was much more workable and usable just at the time of resurgence of interest and community activity in the field.

Some further refinements were added by the clinicians Perlstein, Crothers, and Paine [35,36], which slightly expanded Phelps' approach. Their influence was strong in the subsequent classification prepared by Minear for the American Academy for Cerebral Palsy. In addition to motor types, distribution and degree of involvement as well as extent of treatment required were included for the first time [37].

Physiological (Motor)
   Spasticity
   Athetosis   Tension; nontension; dystonia; tremor
   Rigidity
   Ataxia
   Tremor
   Atonia (rare)
   Mixed
   Unclassified

Distribution

Severity

Treatment

Some ambiguity exists in several of the Minear motor types, for example, the distinction between tremor athetosis and a separate tremor category. How does tremor differ from ataxia? Is there a physiological equivalent of atonia, or is this part of a developmental stage from which one of the other types ultimately emerges? Are some motor patterns unclassifiable again because they represent transient developmental features only?

These questions are relevant because the Minear classification was prepared almost twenty-five years ago when cerebral palsy was diagnosed late and solely on the recognition of a fixed motor deficit type. The developmental characteristics of the condition and especially the emerging nature of the neurological lesion were not appreciated. Depending upon the age at which a child was initially seen, the motor features would be variably evident. A modern classification therefore must consider the early signs of developmental abnormality and the emerging motor type. Such a classification could dispel confusion regarding diagnosis and provide better communication among the various professionals dealing with the child. An attempt is made to develop this approach in Chapter 2.

ETIOLOGICAL CONSIDERATIONS

Congenital Cerebral Palsy

This refers to conditions in which the etiology is traced to intrauterine, natal, or perinatal factors and was estimated by Perlstein to include some eighty-five percent of all cases [21]. The complexity of etiological association to the condition itself and to various motor types was apparent to Little. He recognized that spastic paraplegia was generally associated with a preterm but normal delivery, whereas spastic quadriplegia was more often found with an abnormal term delivery [5].

That prematurity is a major factor in cerebral palsy has subsequently been well-established and is noted in at least one-third of cases (38-46]. The mutlivariate nature of prematurity however, raises serious questions about discrete causal factors and many uncertainties remain to be resolved. Gestational age itself must be considered in addition to birth weight. The small for gestational age (SGA) child appears less likely to have cerebral palsy and more at risk for genetic disorders, mental retardation, and global neurological deficit than the child who is of appropriate weight for gestational age (A.G.A.) [47].

The role of neonatal asphyxia remains controversial among premature births, in spite of frequent respiratory distress syndrome and apnea in this group. Churchill, and Davies and Tizard, for example, found no greater percentage with asphyxia among children less than 2000 grams compared with controls [40,43]

Intracranial hemorrhage, especially among premature babies is well-established and has been related to rupture of a disproportionately large middle cerebral artery. This is given further support in the collaborative cerebral palsy study indicating significant anemia among affected premature babies as the only feature distinguishing them from nonaffected controls [49].

Other aspects suggesting a relation especially to prematurity include intrauterine malnutrition [50] and intrinsic developmental disability of

the fetus [51]. Disproportionate central nervous system maturation among
prematures has also been suggested [52].

Regardless of gestational age or birth weight, the maternal prenatal condition may have a significant effect on subsequent CNS development and
pathology of the fetus. General health status and untreated medical conditions may be relevant. Effects of drugs, alcohol, tobacco, exposure to radi-
ation, or environmental pollutants are all known to have some bearing on
fetal development but the possible relation to cerebral palsy is not established. Factors directly affecting maturation of the placenta are not clear
but could be highly relevant. Maternal infection remains a major source of
fetal CNS pathology. The primary conditions of concern are congenital
rubella, toxoplasmosis, cytomegalovirus, and herpes. Each may be without
serious or even noticeable clinical manifestations during gestation.

Neonatal asphyxia is the most significant perinatal event. This may be related to obstetrical accident, dystocia, anesthesia, nuchal cord or other mechanical problems, or intrinsic pulmonary deficit of the infant [53].

Intracranial hemorrhage appears to be a less likely causative event at
birth for the full-term child. Infection during the perinatal period may be
significant, particularly if it leads to sepsis or meningitis. Hyperbilirubinemia
of the newborn due to Rh factor, ABO, or other blood group incompability
was formerly a major factor in development of kernicterus, milder forms of
athetosis, or mixed forms of cerebral palsy. Its impact has been greatly reduced by improved methods of early identification, better exchange trans-
fusions, but above all, the preventive use of anti-Rh (D) gamma globulin to
immunize the prospective mother immediately after her first pregnancy
[54]. Neonatal jaundice due to sepsis or physiological immaturity of the
liver may still require careful attention.

Malformations of the CNS may be apparent at birth. Those having a bearing on a fixed motor lesion would include hydrocephalus, anencephaly,
encephalocele, and a variety of intracranial structural deficits, such as Sturge-
Weber syndrome, neurofibromatosis, and other phakomatoses. The extent to
which these are remediable early would determine whether permanent residual abnormality exists.

Acquired Cerebral Palsy

Data regarding fixed intracranial lesions with permanent residua which develop beyond the perinatal period are limited. Records of Perlstein's cases suggest approximately fifteen percent [21], although studies of such lesions in
the general population suggest an astonishingly high frequency [55]. The
major categories include CNS infections, intracranial hemorrhage due to
primary vascular accident, or secondary to a thrombosis from a cardiac lesion,

or sickle cell anemia. Late onset or inadequately treated hydrocephalus may be a major factor. Trauma is particularly common once the child begins to walk and develops independence in the preschool period. Neoplastic intracranial lesions are not rare in the early developing years and may be associated with permanent residua [56].

Genetic Cerebral Palsy

A possible hereditary basis for cerebral palsy has been of considerable historic interest and concern. Multiple cases within a given family lend credence to an earlier popular notion suggesting this. However, objective review generally substantiates a pregnancy or birth history which often could explain multiple involvement. Nevertheless, there are well-documented cases of apparent genetically determined lesions of spastic paraplegia, generalized athetosis, and ataxia [57]. A pattern of autosomal dominance is generally seen and may be traceable through several generations. Pathology in the case of spastic paraplegia is a structural deficit in the pyramidal tract in the upper cervical area [58].

TRENDS IN EPIDEMIOLOGY

Incidence and Prevalence

Since the time of John Little there was no reliable information about the extent of cerebral palsy until the resurgence of interest in the middle of this century.

The first major study included the area around Schnectady, New York, in 1949 [59]. Phelps' research followed shortly thereafter and used an estimated prevalence figure of 7 per 100,000 population for all ages [60]. This is an often quoted statistic which is difficult to compare with other studies covering children up to age twenty-one [61]. Comparison can best be made with incidence data. Perlstein's figure of 7 per 1000 live births had been a well-accepted standard [62]. The subsequent studies of Hagberg [63] and Franco suggest a reduction in case incidence of nearly two-thirds up to the present [64]. However, possible increase in severity must be considered [65, 66].

Factors affecting this trend include improved obstetrical management [67] and technological success of increasingly sophisticated perinatal centers [68] especially for premature infants weighing less than 1500 grams [69], and without severe respiratory problems [70]. Reduction in frequency and improved management of maternal infection, particularly rubella, is also significant.

Cerebral Palsy Types and Distribution

Considerable change is also noted in relative frequency of the major cerebral palsy motor types. Spasticity continues to be most common and is generally considered to be present in greater than fifty percent of cases [64]. A considerable reduction is noted now in spastic diplegia (generally associated with prematurity), especially among those weighing more than 1000 grams at birth. Interestingly, little change is noted in frequency of spastic quadriplegia [63]. Athetosis was formerly noted in one-third of cases and has been reduced to ten percent or less [64], largely as a result of both improved treatment and prevention of neonatal byperbilirubinemia.

Ataxia due to a fixed cerebellar lesion is seen in from five to ten percent and appears to be unchanged. Rigidity was thought to comprise about one percent of cases [21]. Current clinical experience suggests it to be a rarely used category. This may reflect a better understanding of developmental neurological deficit; many cases formerly in this category are now more appropriately classified as athetosis with tension or mixed forms.

Mixed types of cerebral palsy also appear to be more commonly identified than previously, and are now probably only second in importance to spasticity. The opportunity for early initial and subsequent long-term observation seems to favor this category increasingly and may give a more accurate picture of the diffuse involvement which can be identified as the central nervous system matures.

Degree of Severity

About one-third of patients have generally been considered to be equally distributed into the mild, moderate, and severely involved categories. Recent review by Franco, however, has indicated (Table 2) considerable differences between premature and full-term infants [64].

The greater degree of profound involvement among premature babies is of significance since this remains a major etiologic category.

Table 2   Degree of Severity of Cerebral Palsy

Degree of Severity	Prematures (%)	Full-Term (%)
Profound	33	20
Moderate	27	36
Slight	40	44

Source: From Ref. 64.

Associated Handicaps

No current studies include specific data on extent of visual, speech, and hearing deficits; seizure disorders; or mental retardation in association with cerebral palsy. However, some inferences can be made using knowledge about current trends in the condition. Less high-frequency hearing loss is probably found since this was seen regularly in athetosis. Both seizure disorders and degree of mental retardation closely parallel severity of cerebral palsy, and will reflect the pattern of greater involvement among very small prematures. A greater recognition of associated severe perceptual–motor and other learning disabilities is now present.

Current Trends

The apparent considerable reduction in overall incidence of cerebral palsy has recently come under critical review [71]. It appears to be selective for those infants formerly subject to events in the immediate perinatal period. Low-weight prematures are now surviving in increasing numbers and are subject to severe developmental risk [72]. Data from Sweden indicating little difference in frequency of spastic quadriplegia support this concept [63]. Current progress in maternal and infant care indeed confirms greater survival of "at risk" children. Survival of those subject to greatest physiological stress is likely to be associated with severe neurological deficit in the form of cerebral palsy [73].

In contrast with Little's day, we are fortunate in having available the techniques for early identification and tools for early intervention which may enable survivors with even severe involvement to develop some independent function and eventually make their contribution to society. This has become possible as the early limited orthopedic approach has increasingly expanded to include multiple professionals, all of whom must deal together with the array of needs of the developmentally disabled.

REFERENCES

1. Cazauvielh, J.: Recherches sur l'agenesie cerebral et la paralysie congeniale. *Arch. Gen Med.* 1827.
2. Delpech, M.: Tenotomie de tendon d'Achilles, In Chiurgeric Clinique de Montpellier, Observations et Reflexions Tirees des Travaux de Chirurgie Clinique de Cette Ecole. Paris, Gabon, 1828, p. 181.
3. Little, W.: Course of lectures on deformation of the human frame. Lecture number VIII. *Lancet* 1:318, 1843.
4. Little, W.: On the Nature and Treatment of the Deformities of the Human Frame. London, Longman, Brown, Green and Longman, 1853.

5. Little, W.: On the influence of abnormal parturition, difficult labours, premature birth, and asphyxia neonatorum on the mental and physical condition of the child, especially in relation to deformities. *Trans. Obstet. Soc. London,* 3:293, 1861.

6. Gowers, W.: On birth palsies. *Lancet* 1:709, 1888.

7. Osler, W.: The Cerebral Palsies of Children: A Clinical Study from the Infirmary for Nervous Diseases. Philadelphia, Blakiston, 1889.

8. Freud, S.: Die infantile cerebrallahmung in Nothnagel, J.: Specialle Pathologie und Therapie, Band IX, Th.III. Vienna, Holder, 1897.

9. Colby, J.: Massage and remedial exercises in the treatment of children's paralysis: Their difficulties in use. *Boston Med. Surg. J.* 173:696, 1915.

10. Lord, E.: Children Handicapped by Cerebral Palsy. New York, Commonwealth Fund, 1937.

11. Stoffel, A.: The treatment of spastic contracture. *Am. J. Orthop. Surg.,* 10:611, 1913.

12. Phelps, W.: The treatment of cerebral palsies. *J. Bone Joint Surg.* 22: 1004, 1940.

13. Wolf, J.: The Results of Treatment in Cerebral Palsy. Springfield, Chas. C Thomas, 1969, pp. 10-11.

14. Vining, E., Accardo, P., Rubenstein, J., Farrell, S., and Roizen, N.: Cerebral palsy: a pediatric developmentalist's overview. *Am. J. Dis. Child.* 130:643, 1976.

15. Katz, A.: Parents of the Handicapped. Springfield, Chas. C Thomas, 1961, p. 23.

16. United Cerebral Palsy. The Story of U.C.P. New York, 1949.

17. Merkatz, I., and Johnson, K.: Regionalization of perinatal care for the United States. *Clin. Perinatol.* 3:271, 1976.

18. Haynes, U.: The First Three Years—Programming for Atypical Infants and Their Families. New York, United Cerebral Palsy Association, 1974.

19. Tjossem, T. D. (Ed.): Intervention Strategies for the High Risk Infant. Baltimore, University Park Press, 1976.

20. Greenspan, L.: The conception, growth and development of the developmentalist. Presidential address. American Academy for Cerebral Palsy and Developmental Medicine, Atlanta, 1977.

21. Perlstein, M.: Infantile cerebral palsy: classification and clinical observations. *JAMA* 149:30, 1952.

22. Burgess, D.: A case of cerebral birth palsy. *Med. Chron. Manchester* 9:471, 1888.

23. Sachs, B., and Peterson, F.: A study of cerebral palsies in early life-based upon an analysis of one hundred and forty cases. *J. Nerv. Ment. Dis.* 17:295, 1890.

24. Brissaud, E.: Maladie de Little et tabes spasmodique. *Sem. Med.* 14: 89, 1894.
25. Rosenberg, L.: Der cerebralen Kinderlähmungen Kassowitz. *Beitr. Kinderheilkd.* Neue Folge IV, 1893.
26. Freud, S., and Rie, C.: Klinische Studien Uber Die Hoslbseitige Cerebral-Lähmung der Kinder, Vienna, Perles, 1891.
27. Phelps, W.: Let's define cerebral palsy. *Crippled Child* 26:4, 1948.
28. O'Reilly, D.: History of the American Academy for Cerebral Palsy and Developmental Medicine. Washington, DC, AACPDM, 1979.
29. Breakey, A.: Ocular findings in cerebral palsy. *Arch. Ophthalmol.* 53:852, 1955.
30. Vernon, m.: Clinical phenomena of cerebral palsy and deafness. *Except. Child.* 36:743, 1970.
31. Robinson, R.: The frequency of other handicaps in children with cerebral palsy. *Dev. Med. Child. Neurol.* 15:305, 1973.
32. Hopkins, T., Bice, H., and Colton, K.: Evaluation and Education of the Cerebral Palsy Child. Washington, D.C., Intl. Council for Exceptional Children, 1954.
33. Fay, T.: Cerebral palsy: medical considerations and classification. *Am. J. Psychiatry* 107:180, 1950.
34. Phelps, W.: Etiology and diagnostic classification of cerebral palsy. In, Proceedings of the Cerebral Palsy Institute. New York, Association for the Aid of Crippled Children, 1950.
35. Perlstein, M.: Medical aspects of cerebral palsy. *Nervous Child* 8:128, 1949.
36. Crothers, B., and Paine, R.: The Natural History of Cerebral Palsy. Cambridge, Harvard Universtiy Press, 1959.
37. Minear, W.: A classification of cerebral palsy. *Pediatrics* 18:841, 1956.
38. Bandera, E., and Churchill, J.: Prematurity and neurological disorders. *Henry Ford Hosp. Med. Bull.* 9:414, 1961.
39. Berenberg, W., and Ong, B.: Cerebral spastic paraplegia and prematurity. *Pediatrics* 33:496, 1964.
40. Churchill, J.: The relationship of Little's disease to premature birth. *Am. J. Dis. Child.* 96:32, 1958.
41. Childs, B., and Evans, P.: Birth weights of children with cerebral palsy. *Lancet* 1:642, 1954.
42. Drillien, C.: Growth and development in a group of children of very low birth weight. *Arch. Dis. Child.* 33:10, 1958.
43. Davies, P., and Tizard, J.: Very low birth weight and subsequent neurological defect. *Dev. Med. Child.* Neurol. 17:3, 1975.
44. Eastman, N., Kohl, S., Maisel, J., and Kavaler, F.: The obstetrical background of 753 cases of cerebral palsy. *Obstet. Gynecol. Surv.* 17:459, 1962.

45. McDonald, A.: Cerebral palsy in children of very low birth weight. *Arch. Dis. Child.* 38:579, 1963.
46. Wright, F., Blough, R., Chamberlin, A., Ernest, T., Halstead, W., Meier, P., Moore, R., Naunton, R., and Newell, F.: A controlled follow up study of small prematures born from 1952 through 1956. *Am. J. Dis. Child.* 124:506, 1972.
47. Scherzer, A., and Mike, V.: Cerebral palsy and the low birth weight child. *Am. J. Dis. Child.* 128:199, 1974.
48. Koenigsberger, R. (Ed.): Symposium on High Risk Pregnancy and High Risk Babies. American Academy for Cerebral Palsy, New York, 1971.
49. Churchill, J., Masland, R., Nagler, A., and Ashworth, M.: The Etiology of Cerebral Palsy in Prematures. American Academy for Cerebral Palsy, New York, 1971.
50. Sabel, K., Olegard, R., and Victoria, L.: Remaining sequelae with modern perinatal care. *Pediatrics* 57:652, 1976.
51. Polani, P.: Prematurity and cerebral palsy. *Br. Med. J.* 2:1497, 1958.
52. Churchill, J.: The relationship of Little's disease to premature birth. *Am. J. Dis. Child.* 96:32, 1958.
53. Roboz, P.: Etiology of congenital cerebral palsy. *Arch. Pediat.* 79: 233, 1962.
54. Spellacy, W. (Ed.): Management of the High Risk Pregnancy. Baltimore, University Park Press, 1976.
55. Schoenberg, B.: The spectrum of cerebrovascular disease in infants and children. Annual meeting, American Academy for Cerebral Palsy and Developmental Medicine. Atlanta, 1977.
56. Matson, D.: Neurosurgery in Infancy and Childhood. Springfield, Chas. C Thomas, 1969.
57. Cooper, W., German, J., and Lame, E.: Genetic implications of cerebral palsy. *J. Bone Joint Surg.* [Am.] 47:1673, 1965.
58. Silver, J.: Familial spastic paraplegia with amyotrophy of the hands. *Ann. Hum. Genet.* 30:69, 1966.
59. Cruickshank, W., and Raus, G.: Cerebral Palsy. Syracuse, Syracuse University Press, 1955.
60. Phelps, W.: Etiology and diagnostic classification of cerebral palsy. In, Proceedings of the Cerebral Palsy Institute, New York, Association for the Aid of Crippled Children, 1950.
61. Henderson, J.: Cerebral Palsy in Childhood. Edinburgh, Livingstone, 1961.
62. Perlstein, M., and Barnett, H.: Nature and recognition of cerebral palsy in infancy. *JAMA* 148:1389, 1952.
63. Hagberg, B., Hagberg, G., and Olow, I.: The changing panorama of cerebral palsy in Sweden 1954-1970. I. Analysis of general changes. *Acta Paediatr. Scand.* 64:187, 1975.

64. Franco, S., and Andrews, B.: Reduction of cerebral palsy by neonatal intensive care. *Pediatr. Clin. North Am.* 24:639, 1977

65. Nelson, K., and Ellenberg, J.: Epidemiology of Cerebral Palsy. In Schoenberg, B. (Ed.): Advances in Neurology. Vol. 19. New York, Raven Press, 1978, pp. 421-435.

66. Kitchen, W., Rickards, A., Ryan, M., McDougall, A., Billson, F., Keir, E., and Naylor, F.: A longitudinal study of very low-birth weight infants. II: results of controlled trial of intensive care and incidence of handicaps. *Dev. Med. Child. Neurol.* 21:582, 1979.

67. Fanaroff, A., and Merkatz, I.: Modern obstetrical management of the low birth weight infant. *Clin. Perinatol.* 4:215, 1977.

68. Fitzhardinge, P., Kalman, E., Ashby, S., and Pape, K.: Present status of the infant of very low birth weight treated in a referral neonatal intensive care unit in 1974. *Ciba Found. Symp.* 59:139, 1978.

69. Steward, A., and Reynolds, E.: Improved prognosis for infants of very low birth weight. Pediatrics 54:724, 1974.

70. Steward, A., Turcan, D., Rawlings, G., Hart, S., and Gregory, S.: Outcome for infants at high risk of major handicap. *Ciba Found. Symp.* 59:151, 1978.

71. Kiely, J., Paneth, N., Stein, Z., and Susser, M.: Cerebral palsy and newborn care. I. Secular trends in cerebral palsy. Devel. Med. Child. Neurol. 23:533, 1981.

72. Kiely, J., Paneth, N., Stein, Z., and Susser, M.: Cerebral palsy and newborn care. II. Mortality and neurological impairment in low-birth weight infants. Devel. Med. Child. Neurol. 23:650, 1981.

73. Paneth, N., Kiely, J., Stein, Z., and Susser, M.: Cerebral palsy and newborn care. III. Estimated prevalence rates of cerebral palsy under differing rates of mortality and impariment of low-birth weight infants. Devel. Med. Child. Neurol. 23:801, 1981.

2
Developmental Evaluation and Differential Diagnosis

THE CONCEPT OF NORMAL
NEUROLOGICAL MATURATION

The work of Gesell and others firmly established both uniformity and the concept of variation in the normal developmental sequence of children [1-3]. Acquaintance with this basic framework is essential to a working understanding of the growth process. More importantly, it is the cornerstone upon which identification and understanding of abnormal development rest. Some general principles of development are helpful in providing an overview.

There is a fairly orderly process from birth which is continuous with in-utero development [4]. The neurophysiological basis of this process is ascending development of brain center control [5]. Initially, newborn infant behavior is largely on a reflex basis, mediated primarily through the brain stem. Maturation then proceeds towards "higher" centers, ultimately reaching independence in full voluntary control. However, it should be noted that some degree of voluntary movement is present even in the neonate. Thus the infantile primitive reflexes give way to more complex postural reflexes and proceed to full voluntary behavior. Also the initial mass behavior activity on a reflex basis is replaced by individual responses under voluntary control.

Motor maturation then proceeds in a cephalocaudal direction: motor control of the head, neck, and trunk preceeds extension of the trunk, ultimate weight bearing, and walking.

Maturation of the normal central nervous system occurs simultaneously at many different levels. Although there is an orderly sequence in development, considerable variation is seen within a given child in achieving stages of motor and intellectual achievement. Thus, a child's intelligence may be considerably ahead of his or her locomotion ability, yet ultimately development may reach normal levels. Acceptable degree of variation exists among infants in reaching established levels of maturation.

Finally, motor development should be seen as a succession of integrated milestones leading to more complex and independent function [6]. Each stage is interdependent and relates closely to progressive control of higher centers of the nervous system and reduced influence of fixed reflex behavior [7]. Many stages will be developing simultaneously. Each milestone, therefore, is not perfected before going on to the next [8]. Also a "competition of motor patterns" is suggested in which a child carries out natural practicing of new activities with temporary suppression of others until learning is complete. Older and more established activities may be then resumed and added [9].

The challenge for those dealing with developmental problems in children is accurately to assess and comprehend the significance of delay which falls outside of the limits of variability. Is it normal or pathological? Knowledge of the normal, the orderly sequence of developmental achievement, and patterns of integration of behavior is the basis upon which possibly significant deviation in maturation can be gauged. Appendix A includes a comprehensive outline of developmental stages and normal motor milestones for detailed reference, from ages two months to two years.

OVERVIEW OF ABNORMAL DEVELOPMENT

While the theme of development is that of a continuum with many variations, its physiological basis is exceedingly complex and does not necessarily coincide with observable function at a given stage in the infant. Growth of nerve pathways, interconnections, and cell fiber proceeds actively to trunk and extremities while brain stem connections and influence remain predominant [10]. Myelination or development of the nerve insulation sheath, for example, is an active process thought, at least, to take up to the first two years before completion [11]. Thus the infant is initially dominated by the primitive reflexes mediated through the brain stem, and by mass response as physical and undoubtedly biochemical growth of the nervous system proceeds. The orderly process leads to gradual inhibition of primitive reflexes, emergence of postural reflex patterns, and increasing voluntary behavior, simultaneously.

Malformation or insult to the central nervous system of the neonate will initially affect brain stem function. Alteration in appearance, intensity, or expression of primitive reflex behavior will result [12]. The normal course of early disappearance of primitive reflexes through inhibition pathways will be affected, with either delay or failure in the development of later postural reflex patterns [13].

Tone will be altered; either excessive or diminished quality will be present. This is mediated through brain stem pathways and will be an early indication of brain stem malfunction [14].

Developmental milestones will be delayed in progression with fixation at a given stage for a prolonged period. The degree of abnormality will relate to the degree of delay in brain stem inhibition and nerve pathway maturation. Both would be directly affected by the nature and degree of the central nervous system fixed pathology.

Motor abnormality of the total nervous system would appear relatively late in development of the infant as nerve pathways become more functional. This is a natural outcome of the selective nerve growth process. Differential rates or order of appearance of motor deficit are manifest. The abnormal motor patterns emerge as the damaged nervous system matures. For example, evidence of specific spasticity may be first noted at seven to nine months of age. Athetosis will not generally be apparent before eighteen months and may be delayed beyond two years. Ataxia is frequently not seen before thirty months to three years. Identification of mixed motor patterns may be further delayed while the nervous system development progresses and relative dominance of one motor form interchanges with another.

The consequences of a fixed lesion of the central nervous system affecting the motor area and development must be seen as emerging and concomitant with growth of the system itself. It is a dynamic, active process, at least from the initial moment of postnatal life and probably earlier. Cerebral palsy is not to be conceived as one or more types of fixed motor disturbance but an array of developmental disorders which may affect the most primitive functions, the most sophisticated voluntary actions, and often both.

Understanding of the broad developmental scope of the condition forms the basis for both identification and intervention. It is no longer acceptable to simply deal with the spastic foot, the athetoid posture, or the ataxic gait. Consideration must be given as early as possible to definite recognition that a global developmental abnormality exists, so that appropriate means can be directed to remediate the spectrum of deficit of the entire nervous system.

DEVELOPMENTAL EVALUATION APPROACH
TO DIAGNOSIS

The complex developmental nature of the condition with late emerging motor signs makes early identification of cerebral palsy a diagnostic challenge. There is obviously no early pathognomonic sign, x-ray, or laboratory test which in itself is confirmatory. Evidence to substantiate a diagnosis must be gathered in an orderly sequential way with full knowledge of the total maturation process rather than fixation on a focal neurological or physical deficit. This is the developmental approach to diagnosis.

One must start with concern about risk and an index of suspicion. The beginning point is often the pediatrician, family practitioner, or other health professional who is consulted by a worried parent whose child is not progressing in motor milestones or speech. Too often the matter may not be given serious consideration if definite focal motor abnormality is not found. The parent may be reassured and told to return if no progress is forthcoming, in the hope that delayed development will ultimately speed up and resume a normal pattern. A similar situation may occur as well in a highly sophisticated neonatal intensive care unit from which an infant is discharged following treatment for respiratory distress syndrome. Difficulty in feeding and ordinary infant management when brought to the attention of medical staff on follow-up clinic visits may be attributed to immaturity, poor organization at home, or emotional upset by the family.

In fact, each of these situations may represent a child with significant developmental delays due to a fixed motor lesion which ultimately will appear as one of the major motor forms of cerebral palsy. Parental concern may well be appropriate while the professional response is dilatory or nonexistent.

Professional awareness is the starting point in early diagnosis and must be based upon a sensitivity to possible neurological deficit in any child with developmental delay or infant behavior problems. The basis of parental concern must be probed further, rather than merely looking for discrete structural or neurological abnormality. Knowledge of the developmental process needs to be incorporated into the professional's function and used appropriately as any other diagnostic tool. Only in this way will it be possible to develop a realistic and appropriate sense of whether a child is in fact at risk of cerebral palsy or other developmental disability. The index of suspicion should then generate initiation of a full process of developmental evaluation—and not physical examination alone. This should be recorded on a form such as that illustrated in Appendix B.

Developmental History

The chief complaint or concern of the parent presents the initial focus. Often, this is diffuse and sometimes disorganized with confusion about the actual problem. "Advice" from friends and relatives, and poorly understood information from the media may greatly color the real issues. The time-consuming procedure of directing and putting into order these concerns may discourage even the most patient examiner. Skillful and well-directed interviewing, however, will channel unrelated or even diffuse information into a pattern which is digestable and able to be integrated into the history to follow. The examiner should elicit not only the area of most concern but the age and circumstances at which the problem was first noted. This will be of help in guiding discussion about the needs of the family.

An accurate and complete history is the first step in the process of developmental evaluation. Adequate records must be obtained where possible. However, birth and hospital records may not be sufficiently detailed or accurate, particularly if obstetrical or neonatal events have been complex or traumatic. On the other hand, reliability and possible bias of the parent or guardian should be weighed in assessing the information given. It is of importance to be well-organized in obtaining information using a logical sequence for questions, so that major gaps or omissions can be reduced. Factors which may be of significance are discussed below.

Family and Genetic History

Parental and sibling health should be reviewed, particularly as it relates to the period before the pregnancy. Endocrine and metabolic disorders such as thyroid, pituitary abnormality, or diabetes may be relevant. History of seizures and other central nervous system (CNS) problems should be detailed. These would include any evidence of previous mental retardation, learning disorders, cerebral palsy, emotional disorders, congenital malformations, or multiple handicapping conditions among any family members. Evidence for any genetic disease should be elicited, particularly possible patterns of genetic developmental transmission. These may include such conditions as Down's syndrome, Sturge-Weber syndrome and related disorders, genetic forms of cerebral palsy, and evidence for familial organic learning disorders or varieties of mental retardation.

Pregnancy

Quality of the pregnancy is important and relates to feeling of well-being or anxiety, presence of bleeding, health problems, and fetal movements. Each of these may give an indication of pertinent abnormality. Persistent bleeding may indicate intrauterine developmental abnormality especially if it occurred early. Infection, toxemia, and use of medication such as diuretics, anticonvulsants, and various types of antibiotics may be of importance. Late onset or diminished fetal movement may indicate a poorly developing fetus. History of possible trauma or stress should be carefully evaluated.

Length of gestation and the presence of prematurity may be crucial. It is often difficult to obtain an accurate history of pregnancy length due to conflicting dates and various obstetrical calculation methods. Every effort should be made to document possible premature gestation to assess better the relation to birth weight and the extent of developmental risk.

Labor and Delivery

Details of labor should include extent of labor before delivery and rate of progression. Evidence for dystocia or prolonged labor should be considered as well as precipitate or rapid labor. Either may be of considerable significance. A prolonged period between membrane rupture and delivery could be a basis for fetal infection. Obstetrical features of the delivery must include use of anesthesia, mechanical events such as version, abnormal presentations, use of instrumentation, and rationale for caesarean section if performed. The place of delivery may be relevant, especially if at home, en route to the hospital, or under unusual circumstances.

Perinatal and Neonatal Events

Assessment of condition of the child at birth requires information about birth weight, presence of a nuchal cord, respiratory status, the need for prolonged oxygen treatment, continuous apnea, cyanosis, or resuscitative procedures. History is needed of possible sepsis, meningitis, neonatal seizures, and the presence of any type of congenital malformation. Jaundice shortly after birth due to possible blood group incompatibility should be distinguished from subsequent byperbilirubinemia in the neonatal period possibly related to breast feeding, galactosemia, infection such as hepatitis, or structural abnormality of the liver.

History of progress up to the first month should be selectively examined for an overview of the entire neonatal period. Particular attention is needed to review activity and behavior of the infant, looking for evidence of marked irritability, hyperactivity, limited environmental contact, or interaction with the environment. Feeding activity may be crucial, especially if the child sucks or swallows poorly and is thought to have "colic." This may be one of the earliest signs of central nervous system malfunction.

Developmental Milestones

The major developmental milestones present an orderly sequence through which the child is expected to progress normally. An arrest or delay at a given stage is usually the basis for initial parental referral. Not uncommonly, this is the reference point from which the examiner must go back and bring into focus a chief complaint as a first step in the developmental evaluation process.

A table of milestones with variation is given in Appendix A. It is useful to elicit this information in the following order, specifically inquiring about when each of the modalities was achieved: (a) smiling; (b) head control in prone position; (c) grasping; (d) transferring; (e) sitting; (f) crawling including quality of motion; (g) independent walking with quality of movement and evidence of any deficits.

Oral development should be carefully reviewed including any difficulties in sucking, chewing, tongue thrusting, and drooling; problems in both eruption, enamelization, or jaw structure, and dental development. Onset of speech should be noted, including intelligibility and quality of sounds, with a description of progression to phrases and sentences. Verbal behavior is most important, bearing in mind verbosity, repetitive speech, and early evidence of echolalia. Information should also be obtained about hearing acuity and discrimination, visual development, and the onset of and response to environmental stimuli.

The developmental milestones present the major clinical parameter of progressive central nervous system growth and integration. Delay or arrest beyond the normally acceptable range may provide the most significant confirmatory evidence of developmental disability, particularly when considered in conjunction with abnormality in family background, pregnancy, labor, or delivery. No one factor alone will necessarily be definitive but all taken together will form a framework to establish the diagnosis.

Table 1 illustrates the significance of developmental milestones contrasting a normal with a cerebral palsy population. Note the wide range of normal appearance in each modality and a very marked delay among the cerebral palsy group.

Other Developmental Features

Social and emotional variables give an insight into personality integration. Attention should be given to temper tantrums, breath-holding, hyperactivity, limited attention span, and ability to separate from family and adjust in new situations. Play interests are important and should be appropriate for age. These will closely correlate with any obvious physical deficits or limitations. Reaction to and participation in group activities such as preschool or nursery

Table 1 Normal Development Compared with Average Development of 100 Cerebral Palsy Children

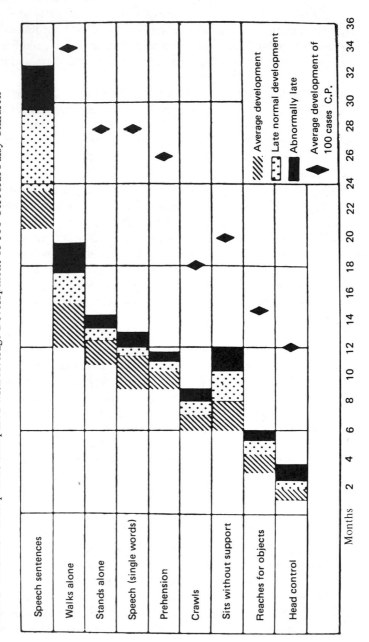

Source: Courtesy of Crippled Children and Adults of Rhode Island, Inc., Providence, Rhode Island

classes gives an insight into demands for attention, supervision, ability to react both physically and socially. Independence in self-care activities should be assessed. These include feeding, undressing and dressing, and toileting. Problems with the latter may have both neurological and emotional aspects which should be carefully weighed. Finally, nursery and preschool adjustment and function will provide an early indication of behavioral problems, learning disabilities, or fine motor function, and should be noted.

Review of Systems

Obviously, particular consideration should be given to general medical or health problems, either associated with or related to possible neurological deficit. Examples would include headaches, unexplained vomiting, lethargy, personality change, or loss of previously achieved function. Any of these could be related to hydrocephalus, an intracranial vascular lesion, or neoplasm. Details of any seizure activity should include whether or not they were associated with fever, frequency, duration, and character of the movements. The history must indicate details of previous neurological evaluation with description of electroencephalogram and other findings, drugs utilized, and results.

Past Medical History

Apart from seizure history, information should include data from any previous neurological, psychological, and developmental evaluations for which appropriate medical records should be obtained. Documentation of medications in use should include rationale and effect. Previous treatment including occupational, physical, and speech therapies should be noted with details of associated changes and the child's response. Similar data is needed about bracing procedures or assistive devices used and types of surgery performed.

At the conclusion of the developmental history, the examiner should indicate an impression of parental interest, attitude, and ability to deal with the child. During the course of the interview it is generally possible to arrive at some awareness of these interpersonal factors which can later provide a basis for needed supportive services.

The Developmental Physical Examination

The setting of the examination is important and should provide a relaxed, unhurried atmosphere for parent and child. Obtained measurements of height, weight, and head circumference should be plotted on appropriate standards and analyzed. The Nellhaus scales of head circumference should be regularly employed as the most accurate measurement [15].

Observation of the child gives the first indication of environmental response, social interaction, and relation to parent. Much of this can be done while the developmental history is obtained. Evidence should be noted for possible visual or hearing deficits, and the quality of verbal response or speech. Level and appropriateness of activity and behavior can also be gauged.

Structural abnormalities must be detailed in an orderly manner through examination of skin, head and neck, trunk, abdomen, back, spine, and extremities. Obvious malformations could immediately identify such conditions as Down's syndrome, Sturge-Weber syndrome, neurofibromatosis, tuberous sclerosis, hydrocephalus, meningomyelocele, encephalocele, hemiplegia, and brachial plexus paralysis [16]. Many other minor structural deviations may also be apparent early. Some may be part of a syndrome complex such as abnormal facial features in fetal alcohol syndrome. Others more frequently will not form part of a specific classification but their presence may suggest associated central nervous system malformation.

Examination of the head and neck should check for size and shape of fontanelles, cleft palate or lip, structural problems of tongue, mouth, and jaw, and abnormal set or configuration of the ears. This is not unusual in children with multiple anomalies and severe developmental deficit.

Examination of the eyes is not as difficult in small children as might be anticipated if the parent assists. The procedure may be most rewarding. Readily obtainable peripheral eye findings may include strabismus, hypertelorism, epicanthus, cataracts, congenital glaucoma, heterochromia, corneal ring (Wilson's disease), depigmented iris of albinism, blue sclerae of osteogenesis imperfecta, scleral pigmentary deposits with ochronosis, or a cloudy cornea noted in mucopolysaccharidosis.

The fundi must be carefully examined for evidence of retinal inflammation as in rubella, toxoplasmosis, or cytomegalovirus infections. Retinal degeneration may indicate a nonspecific degenerative condition, or retinitis pigmentosa, while macular degeneration is specific for Tay-Sachs disease, Nieman-Pick disease, and Gaucher's disease. Also to be noted are retinal changes indicative of intracranial pressure due to hydrocephalus or tumor, and evidence of possible vascular lesions or malformation.

Neck examination should consider signs of webbing and shortening associated with Klippel-Feil syndrome, platybasia and basilar impression, or possible Turner's syndrome. Congenital torticollis is seen in conjunction with other anomalies, and enlarged thyroid is of major concern. Also, a check should be made for bruits both in the neck and head, for vascular malformations.

Chest evaluation should consider anomalies of the bony thorax such as pectus excavatum and carinium, absent ribs, or aplasia of the pectoralis muscles. Lungs and heart should be assessed for normal functioning.

Abdominal fullness or asymmetry may suggest hydronephrosis associated with renal anomalies, Wilms' tumor, or neuroblastoma. Enlarged liver or spleen would give rise to many diagnostic considerations relating to developmental abnormality including biliary atresia, galactosemia, or Wilson's disease; hemoglobinopathy such as in sickle cell anemia or thalassemia, or congenital red cell abnormality in spherocytosis. Hernia is a common finding, often seen in connection with other malformations.

Genitalia should be noted for ambiguity, abnormality in size or shape, testicular descent, presence of hypo- or epispadius. Evidence of precocious puberty may indicate an intracranial lesion or endocrine malfunction.

Extremities should be examined for poly- or syndactyly, abnormal palmar creases seen in Down syndrome, shortening or asymmetry present in hemiplegia or hemihypertrophy. The hips must be carefully assessed for possible dislocation.

Observation of the back should check for lumbosacral hemangioma, anomalous hair, dermal sinus, or raised lesion consistent with meningomyelocele. Spinal deviation including fixed scoliosis, kyphosis, or excessive lordosis needs further review.

Developmental Neurological Examination

The child's activity in relating to the environment is the point of departure. This may be assessed during the physical examination, special emphasis being given to awareness, interest in the environment and examiner, irritability, attention span, and evidence for hyperactivity. Observation of gross motor function and posture can also be done simultaneously and should include head, neck, and trunk control; sitting; crawling; standing; walking; and hand use. Patterns of movement will indicate the presence of asymmetry consistent with hemiplegia, or excessive involvement on one side, restricted movement in spasticity, or excessive movement in dystonia. Character of the cry, voice, and quality of speech are also readily apparent.

Tone should be assessed early in the examination when the child is most relaxed. Distinction should be made between tone of extremities and trunk and any disparity noted. A pattern of hypertonic extremities with hypotonicity of the trunk may be an indication of underlying dystonia which will emerge as athetosis. The ability of a newborn to dorsiflex the foot onto the shin is considered normal and any restriction may suggest excessive abnormal tone [Ref. 17 and (Fig. 1)]. Degree of head lag has been quantitated as a standardized reference for comparison with the norm [18]. Maintenance of hyperextended trunk and standing with support in the very young infant may be the earliest indication of pathological hypertonus. The floppy child seems to have relatively little control or influence of one joint upon another. Such a

Figure 1 A normal newborn can dorsiflex the foot right onto the shin (from Ref. 4, © 1966, the Williams & Wilkins Co., Baltimore).

finding raises the possibility of a wide differential diagnosis including mental retardation, cerebral palsy, and varieties of myopathies. Generally, children who are extremely hypertonic early and who show an ultimate cerebral palsy diagnosis may eventually have the athetoid form, while those with initial hypotonia may later become spastic [19].

Reflex behavior provides a major assessment of brain stem function and may provide the earliest indication of fixed motor deficit consistent with cerebral palsy long before any discrete motor signs are present. Two major categories function dynamically as the nervous system develops toward maturation of higher centers. The first is a group of *primitive reflexes* present at birth and without which the infant would not be viable. These normally disappear by four to six months with maturation as the *postural reflexes* become manifest. The latter are closely associated with and underlie rolling, sitting, crawling, and walking.

The major primitive reflexes include startle reflex, Moro reflex, rooting, sucking, truncal incurvation, asymmetrical tonic neck reflex, crossed extension, tonic labyrinthine reflex, and others. Diagnostic features and assessment are discussed in detail in Chapters 4 and 5.

Since a large number of primitive reflexes are present, there is controversy concerning which have the greatest clinical meaning and predictive significance. Dagarssies places relatively little importance upon truncal incurvation but considers crossed extension to be critical in maturation [12]. Capute et al., on the other hand, include trunkal incurvation as one of the major predictive reflexes being intensely evaluated in an extensive long-range study [20].

Our own clinical experience has led us to give major consideration to the following primitive reflexes in the diagnostic evaluation: startle, Moro, palmar grasp, rooting, sucking, and asymmetric tonic neck (Fig. 2a–2e). Any persisting beyond four to six months would provide a strong index of suspicion for significant fixed motor brain deficit—particularly in association with an abnormal developmental history. A strong asymmetric tonic neck reflex (ATNR) is always abnormal especially if the child cries in this position. A strong and persistent ATNR is frequently later associated with athetoid cerebral palsy [21].

A number of postural reflexes are also identified whose diagnostic significance is yet to be fully established. Among those found to be clinically relevant are neck righting, parachute or protective extension and the Landau reflex [Fig. 3a and (Ref. 31); Fig. 3b and (Ref. 23)]. These are examined in detail in Chapter 4. An overview of developmental reflex behavior is shown in Table 2, including the pattern of disappearance of the primitive reflexes and appearance of postural reflexes. Each of these should be tested during the diagnostic evaluation and considered in relation to timing, strength of expression, and symmetry.

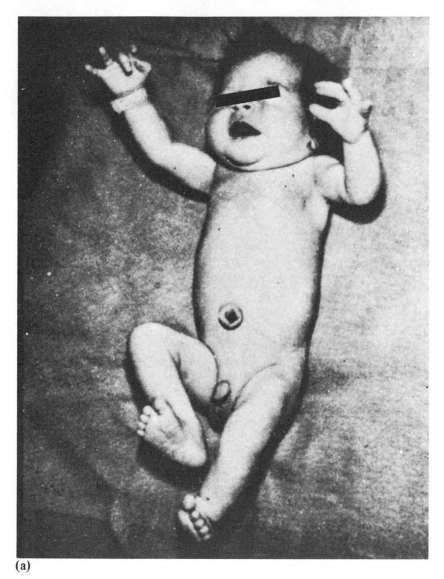

(a)

Figure 2 Primitive reflexes that persist beyond four to six months which may indicate fixed motor brain deficiency: (a) Moro reflex; (b) Palmar grasp reflex. (a and b from Ref. 4, © 1966, The Williams & Wilkins Co., Baltimore.)

(b)

Sensory modalities should include response to touch and pain. Where indicated, specific responses at various dermatome levels should be obtained as in possible lower motor lesions.

Cranial nerve evaluation may be difficult in small children. From a developmental point of view an accurate observation of III, IV, and VI can be obtained for evidence of strabismus; V for mandibular function, and with VII for corneal reflex; VII for facial asymmetry; XI and X for swallowing and gag reflex; XII function may be possible to estimate especially if there is tongue deviation.

Cerebellar dysfunction may be equally difficult to recognize in the infant and very small child. Exaggerated opticokinetic nystagmus should be elicited using response to horizontal movements. Ataxia may be indicated through observation of balance of head, neck, and trunk, and demonstration of hand use with small objects.

(c)

Figure 2 (Continued)   Primitive reflexes that persist beyond four to six months which may indicate fixed motor brain deficiency: (c) rooting reflex; (d) suckling reflex (c–e from Ref. 31).

(d)

Dystonia is often subtle and difficult to identify. Disparity of tone between trunk and extremities may be the first suggestive sign, particularly if
there is significant hypotonicity of the trunk. This may quickly alternate to
truncal hypertonicity. Stiffness and hyperextension of the entire body, but
particularly of the face, head, and upper limbs, may dramatically change.
Apparent limitation in range of motion in the extremities may give way to
full movement and no restriction if the child can be relaxed. In the slightly
older patient facial movements and grimacing may be observed together
with movements of the upper limbs and an overpronated position of arms
and hands. Variable tone remains a cardinal feature which may involve trunk
and extremities. Depending upon the state of the child these features may
vary from time to time, especially in early developmental stages. Actual dys-
tonic movement characteristic of athetosis is likely to appear very late,
whereas the early stiffness judged too rapidly before the child is relaxed is
often misdiagnosed as spasticity. Variability in findings related to athetosis
has also played a part in the past confusion of cerebral palsy classification
(see Chap. 1) particularly relating to "types" of athetosis, and the relation

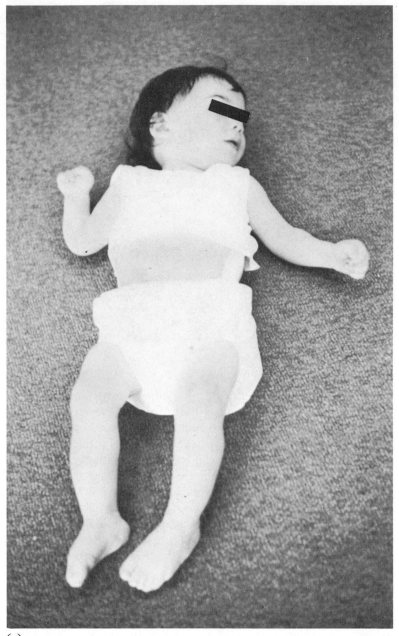

(e)

Figure 2 (Continued) Primitive reflexes that persist beyond four to six months which may indicate fixed motor brain deficiency: (e) Abnormally delayed ATNR).

Table 2 Infant Reflexes and Age (Month) Normally Demonstrated

Months	1	2	3	4	6	9	12	15	18	24
Primitive										
Moro	+	+	±	±	0	0	0	0	0	0
Palmar	+	+	±	±	0	0	0	0	0	0
ATNR	+	+	±	±	0	0	0	0	0	0
Rooting/suck	+	+	+	±	±	0	0	0	0	0
Postural										
Neck right	0	0	0	±	±	+	+	+	+	+
Parachute	0	0	0	0	±	+	+	+	+	+
Landau	0	0	0	0	0	0	+	+	+	±

to the tremor, atonia, rigidity, and even ataxia. The clinical distinction between these can be most difficult in a very small child.

Upper motor neuron signs relating to the motor area and pyramidal tracts can generally be elicited without difficulty, particularly if there is asymmetry. Markedly exaggerated deep tendon reflexes can be judged accurately indicating evidence for spasticity. Babinski sign may be variable and often cannot be definitely evaluated. Its significance even in newborns is also questioned since it may not be found at all [22]. Frequently, clonus can best be demonstrated by placing the child in the prone position and gently dorsiflexing the great toe or anterior part of the foot. This maneuver tends to displace voluntary motor activity away from the feet so that the reflex is not dampened.

Soft signs refer to a group of functional neurological findings which are general and not focal, obten subtle, and may relate to integration in development [23]. They give clues to underlying central nervous system deficit. One of the earliest may affect sucking, swallowing, and feeding and has already been mentioned in connection with neonatal "colic." Persistent irritability, demanding behavior, continuous gross movement and activity, markedly limited attention span, delayed speech with poor or repetitive expression, withdrawn and isolated behavior, irregular sleep habits, may all suggest underlying deficit. A systematic approach to observing others is indicated during examination if the child is capable of some cooperation. These would include visual tracking without moving the head, blowing out the cheeks, demonstrating fine finger movements, rapid succession movements, and at a later stage identifying lateral parts of the body, i.e., right hand, left eye.

The soft signs add another dimension to the diagnostic capability by either confirming impressions from other positive motor findings or suggesting areas

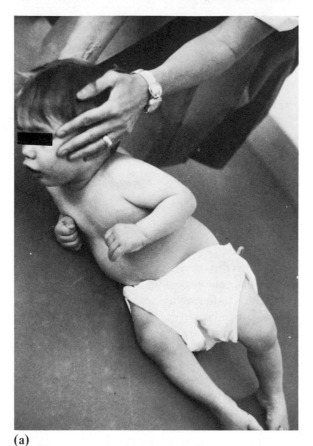

(a)

Figure 3 Postural reflexes of diagnostic and prognostic significance: (a) neck righting reflex; (b) the Landau reflex. (a) from Ref. 31; and (b) from R. S. Paine, Neurological examination of infants and children. (*Pediatr. Clin. North Am.* 7:471, 1960).

other than gross motor as sources of developmental deficit. These might include mental retardation, minimal brain dysfunction, autism, or emotional disorder. More specifically directed diagnostic assessments could then be undertaken.

Screening estimates of psychological functioning are an important aspect of the initial developmental evaluation. Various professionals other than the psychologist can undertake or supplement this function. The Denver Developmental Screening Test is easily administered in a short time by the physician or other professional, and provides a visually descriptive index of

(b)

functioning in fine and gross motor, language, and social skills [24]. It has the added advantage of being easily updated and provides a visual impression of change.

For the older child who is capable of using paper and pencil, a figure copy test is useful to give gross estimates of developmental levels, perceptual motor deficits, ability to follow directions, and degree of attention span. A modified figure copy test with levels of function is given in Appendix C.

The Goodenough test, in which the child of three or older is directed to draw a person may also be administered [25]. This provides an indication of developmental level and may also provide some insights into personality integration. Like the figure copy test, it has the advantage of being easily administered during the developmental examination by the physician or other health personnel.

The Scope of Laboratory Evaluation

The extent to which laboratory procedures are needed to aid in diagnosis will depend upon findings of the physical and neurological examinations in relation to the developmental history. In the child with a history of prematurity and neonatal anoxia who is markedly delayed in milestones and has signs of generalized spasticity, relatively few laboratory data are needed to support a diagnosis of cerebral palsy or spastic quadriplegia. However, a patient who has a normal birth history and marked progressive developmental delay with a paucity of findings, would require hospitalization for an extensive work-up. Considerable variation generally exists in the average case. A major benefit of an organized, sequential system of developmental evaluation is that it provides a focus and direction in the usual office or clinic setting which will help to determine the extent to which more detailed work-up will be indicated. The child with a developmental delay must not be the subject of a shot-gun approach using laboratory findings to determine whether a lesion exists. Rather, the dynamic and changing nature of the central nervous system, especially one in which there is some deficit, has to be viewed in its entirety.

Screening tests which may be useful initially include complete blood count and urinalysis, serum lead levels, T4 for thyroid function, urinary amino acid study, and skull x-rays for evidence of intracranial calcification. Even these procedures should be limited unless clinically indicated.

The electroencephalogram is much abused and frequently misused. It is clearly indicated and should be mandatory where there is a seizure history and may be of considerable assistance in management. Where there is behavior disorder or hyperactivity, it generally has little to add. As a routine procedure it has no place and should be discouraged. Unfortunately, it has come to be regarded as the major developmental diagnostic tool by many teachers and others who deal professionally with children. They often need guidance and direction to discourage this approach. A similar situation seems to be emerging with computerized axial tomography (CAT scan). This highly effective procedure may be vital in the work-up of a child with significant developmental delays. However, its use must be first based upon considerations derived from an orderly sequential approach.

FORMULATING THE DIAGNOSIS

As pointed out earlier, the very young child with a fixed motor lesion will not show focal signs of spasticity, athetosis, ataxia, or combinations. Rather, there will initially be abnormalities of tone, excess of primitive reflex activity with delay in disappearance, and late, often incomplete, emergence of postural reflexes. Developmental history is crucial in diagnosis. Paucity of laboratory findings is to be expected. Where the developmental history is strongly positive and signs of abnormal tone and reflex behavior are present a probable diagnosis of cerebral palsy is appropriate. Utilizing this sequential developmental evaluation procedure will allow a definite diagnosis within the first few months of life and a presumptive one even earlier.

In the older child, generally beyond one year, a diagnosis of cerebral palsy can often be made indicating a specific motor type. This may change as the child grows and the definitive motor defect becomes more apparent. Definitive motor signs may also disappear early in very mild cases. As the child grows, it is possible to formulate specifics of extent and degree of involvement, i.e., cerebral palsy, spastic quadriplegia, mild uppers involvement, moderate lower body involvement. Where possible, it is useful to include these features in the diagnosis so that some outlook for prognosis is available.

It is not always either practical or desirable to place a diagnostic label on a child. When dealing with the very young nervous system, it is often not possible to have complete assurance that developmental history and physical and neurological evaluations are compatible with cerebral palsy, or other specific recognizable entity. However, evidence for definite and significant developmental delay may be present and the judgment or maturity of the examiner will then determine the subsequent course. It is at this point that parents not infrequently are told that the child will "grow out of it." Unfortunately, the outcome is likely to confirm the initial impression of specific pathology. This is particularly true if the systematic process of developmental evaluation is followed.

An examiner is sometimes hesitant to inform parents of possible deficit because treatment or intervention is either not possible or available for the very young child. The rapid rise of early intervention programs and increasing evidence of significant effect for child and family (see Chap. 9) are compelling and should put this approach to rest.

Practitioners may be concerned about unduly alarming parents, believing that a gradual approach over time will be less distressing. Perhaps in time the parents will see for themselves that the child is abnormal and seek help. To be guided by either of these possibilities places the family in severe emotional jeopardy. They are already concerned or would not have come for the evaluation. Without guidance and direction they are likely to seek other opinions and will face further uncertainty and confusion from "shopping around" and obtaining a variety of judgments. Too often, this leads to severe emotional conflict and major adjustment problems within a family.

When some doubt exists about an exact diagnosis or confirmation of cerebral palsy cannot be made with certainty it is best to inform parents that the child shows definite developmental delay without using a specific label. This sets the stage for future action. It may confirm what the parents know already and return balance and stability to the family. A plan of action is decided upon and should include referral for some form of early intervention program. It also keeps open possibilities for future development and demands that the child be seen at regular periodic intervals to monitor change. Continuity of follow-up by the same professional group is essential if at all practical to assess needs and progress fully. Only in this way will it be possible to

Table 3 Early Developmental Deficit Classification

1. Normal child—mild developmental immaturity
2. Developmental delay
   a. Motor
   b. Oral
   c. Psychological
   d. Behavior
3. Developmental abnormality—nonspecific
   a. Motor
   b. Oral
   c. Psychological
   d. Behavior (severity)
      1. Mild
      2. Moderate
      3. Profound

provide adequate communication with and support for parents and plan appropriately for the future. The need for continuous reevaluation does not cease even when a specific diagnosis of a cerebral palsy type can be made. Cerebral palsy is always a presumptive diagnosis since confirmatory evidence is indirect and is based upon behavior and development at a given time. One must always be on guard for any changes which may be consistent with progressive disease, however subtle or slow in nature. This is particularly true of cerebellar or mixed cerebral palsy lesions.

Some classification other than static encephalopathy is helpful to characterize the dynamic and changing developmental deficit which is identified early before a specific diagnosis is possible. The categories in Table 3 are suggested for use with the young child. Such a classification could provide uniformity in description and greatly improve interprofessional communication.

Categories 2 and 3 would require referral for an intervention program and continuous reevaluation. Many would subsequently be placed in a cerebral palsy or other specific diagnostic category.

The recognition of significant developmental deficit in the young child will lead to planning an appropriate program (see Chap. 3). This should be twofold. The first consideration is management: to develop specific techniques and procedures in caring for the child. These are necessary because deficits may severely limit and require alteration of the usual child-care regime. Second, simultaneous treatment or therapy is instituted to guide and stimulate a more normal pattern of neurological development and growth. Both management and treatment constitute the early intervention program which can be offered for the infant with a nonspecific developmental deficit diagnosis as well as the young child with specifically identified cerebral palsy. The process should be continuous and flexible in dealing with the neurological lesion as it becomes increasingly apparent and discrete.

DIFFERENTIAL DIAGNOSTIC CONSIDERATIONS

Nonprogressive Developmental Deficits

Congenital cerebral palsy may be distinguished very early from all other static encephalopathies by the marked immaturity of premature reflex patterns and their late disappearance [26]. This is particularly true if there is prominent and persistent startle, Moro, and obligatory ATNR. Postural reflexes are greatly delayed in cerebral palsy and may, in fact, never develop with any degree of maturity as the discrete motor abnormality evolves.

Acquired cerebral palsy will be identified by specific fixed motor type in a child who had previously been normal and after a specific brain insult. Preceeding features of tone, primitive or postural reflex behavior, and milestones all would have been appropriate.

Few data are available concerning the rare cases of genetic cerebral palsy. In contrast with congenital types, tone and primitive reflexes are nearer normal, while there is delay in postural reflexes and specific abnormality in milestones, i.e., delayed or absent walking in familial spastic paraplegia. There may be a family history of similar cases [27]. In mental retardation syndromes the primitive reflexes are appropriate in expression and disappearance. However, the postural reflexes will develop very late and there will be a significant delay in developmental milestones. This is the major differential point [28].

Minimal brain dysfunction may be characterized by early irritability, continuous demanding behavior, and marked activity. Both primitive and postural reflexes will be normal in development. Milestones may be appropriate or even advanced with the exception of speech which may be greatly delayed in appearance or markedly immature in early maturation.

Sometimes the child with organic brain syndrome is withdrawn and shows autisticlike qualities, having little contact socially or interpersonally. Under these circumstances it is often difficult to differentiate developmental levels or achievement of milestones.

This is equally true of the child with primary emotional disorder. Here the tested reflex behavior would be appropriate. Milestones will be delayed, particularly involving speech.

Progressive CNS Disease

Tumors or vascular malformation must be given serious consideration when the history is normal, no abnormalities are found on examination, yet there is marked abnormality or delay in reflex behavior and milestones. This would be particularly true if earlier milestones had been normal. Hydrocephalus with persistent increased intracranial pressure should be seriously considered in children with full, open fontanelles and a markedly enlarged cranial circumference.

The progressive lipoidoses would be evident by the cherry red macula in Tay-Sachs and Niemann-Pick diseases, and hyperpigmented yellow retinal lesions in Gaucher's disease. Cloudy cornea may be seen in mucopolysaccharidoses, corneal ring in Wilson's disease, and blue sclerae in osteogenesis imperfecta. Primitive and postural reflexes have not been well-studied in these cases but would vary considerably with degree of involvement. All would show delay in appearance of postural reflexes and milestones.

Lesch-Nyhan syndrome occurs in boys in association with high uric acid levels and a specific enzyme defect [29]. Positive family history is frequently noted. Unexplained high fevers are present and severe self-mutilation develops early. Without restraint, amputation of fingers will occur. At twelve to eighteen months typical severe generalized athetosis appears and has been frequently diagnosed as the congenital variety. Unfortunately in this instance the condition is progressive with a grave prognosis.

Other nonspecific progressive disorders of grey or white matter should be considered where the history is normal in association with marked developmental delay. Pelizaeus-Merzbacher disease and a variety of leukodystrophies will be arrived at by exclusion. Alexander's disease is identified by progressive macrocephaly without increased intracranial pressure.

Neuropathies are rare in young children and generally would not be a differential consideration. An infectious polyneuritis with significant functional residua could be considered when onset is acute and infection can be documented. Anterior horn cell infection as in poliomyelitis is generally identifiable without difficulty. Degeneration of the anterior horn cell as in Werdnig-Hoffmann disease or variants would be extremely rare, but should be considered.

Myopathies

A spectrum of benign intrinsic muscle disease is now recognized which may be seen in association with the "floppy child" and delayed milestones. These include nemaline myopathy, central core disease, and others [30]. The outcome is generally favorable.

Muscular dystrophy might be a serious consideration in boys beyond the toddler stage who show delay in progression or actual regression in gross motor development. Abnormality in previous reflex behavior or tone would not be expected.

Myasthenia gravis with severe hypotonia may be seen transiently in newborns in association with maternal disease or may be present as a primary disease. The life-threatening nature of the condition is likely to lead to prompt and extensive evaluation.

Appendix A Child Development from 2 Months Through 2 Years[a]

2 months
    Hands predominantly fisted
    Lifts head up for several seconds while prone
    Startles to loud noise
    Follows with eyes and head over 90 degree arc
    Smiles responsively
    Begins to vocalize single vowel sounds

3 months
    Hands occasionally fisted
    Lifts head up above body plane and holds position
    Holds an object briefly when placed in hand
    Turns head toward object, fixes and follows fully in all directions with eyes
    Smiles and vocalizes when talked to
    Watches own hands, stares at faces
    Laughs

4 months
    Holds head steady while in sitting position
    Reaches for an object, grasps it, brings it to mouth
    Turns head in direction of sound
    Smiles spontaneously

5 to 6 months
    Lifts head while supine
    Rolls from prone to supine
    Lifts head and chest up in prone position
    No head lag
    Transfers object from hand to hand
    Babbles
    Sits with support
    Localizes direction of sound

[a]Represents the age at which the average child acquires the skill.

7 to 8 months
  Sits in tripod fashion without support
  Stands briefly with support
  Bangs object on table
  Reaches out for people
  Mouths all objects
  Says da-da, ba-ba

9 to 10 months
  Sits well without support, pulls self to sit
  Stands holding on
  Waves "bye-bye"
  Drinks from cup with assistance

11 to 12 months
  Walks holding on
  Pincer grasp
  Two to four words with meaning
  Creeps well
  Assists in dressing
  Understands a few simple commands

13 to 15 months
  Walks by self—falls easily
  Says several words, uses jargon
  Scribbles with crayon
  Points to things wanted

18 months
  Climbs stairs holding on, climbs up on chair
  Throws ball
  Builds two to four block tower
  Feed self
  Takes off clothes
  Points to two to three body parts
  Many intelligible words

24 months
  Runs, walks up and down stairs alone (both feet per step)
  Two to three word sentences
  Turns single pages of book
  Builds tower of four to six blocks
  Kicks ball
  Uses pronouns "you," "me," "I"

Source: S. B. Brown. The neurologic examination during the first 2 years of life. In. K.F. Swaiman and F. S. Wright, The Practice of Pediatric Neurology. St. Louis, The C. V. Mosby Co., 1975. Data from Refs. 1 and 4.

Appendix B   Initial Developmental Evaluation: Developmental History

---

Date Completed   Informant:

1. Reason for referral: Reliability:
   Age Disability Recognized and Symptoms Noted

2. Family and Genetic History:

3. Pregnancy History:

4. Labor and Delivery:

5. Perinatal and Neonatal Events:
   a. Condition at birth
   b. Neonatal history

6. Developmental Milestones:
   a. Head balance and control
   b. Smiling
   c. Grasping
   d. Transferring
   e. Rolling
   f. Sitting
   g. Crawling
   h. Walking
   i. Hand preference
   j. Oral development
      1. Feeding and sucking
      2. Tongue and mouth problems
      3. Speech
      4. Dental development
   k. Hearing
   l. Vision

7. Other Developmental Features:
   a. Social
   b. Emotional
   c. Play interests
   d. Self care
      1. Feeding
      2. Dressing
      3. Toileting
   e. School

8. Review of Systems:

Appendix B (Continued)

9. Past Medical History
   a. Previous evaluations
   b. Medication
   c. Therapy
   d. Braces/equipment
   e. Surgery
10. Parental Attitude and Information:

Appendix C Developmental Ages

Figure Copying

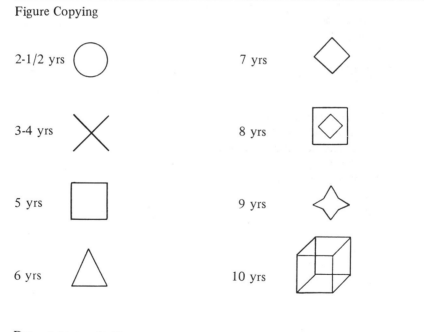

2-1/2 yrs

3-4 yrs

5 yrs

6 yrs

7 yrs

8 yrs

9 yrs

10 yrs

Draw a person test:

REFERENCES

1. Gesell, A., and Amatruda, C.: Developmental Diagnosis, Normal and Abnormal Child Development, Clinical Methods and Pediatric Applications. New York, Hoeber, 1947.
2. Pascal, G., and Jenkins, W.: Systemic Observations of Gross Human Behavior. New York, Grune and Stratton, 1961.
3. Bayley, N.: Value and limitations of infant testing. *Children* 5:129, 1958.
4. Illingworth, R.: The Development of the Infant and Young Child—Normal and Abnormal. Baltimore, Williams & Wilkins, 1966.
5. Jackson, J.: Evolution and dissolution of the nervous system. In Taylor, J. (Ed.): Selected Writings of John Hughlings Jackson. Vol. 2. New York, Basic Books, 1958.
6. Bobath, K.: The Motor Deficit in Patients with Cerebral Palsy. Clinics in Developmental Medicine. London, Heinemann, 1966.
7. Peyser, A.: Cerebral Function in Infancy and Childhood. New York, Consultants Bureau, 1963.
8. Prechtl, H., and Beintema, D.: Neurological Examination of the Full Term Infant. Little Club Clinics in Developmental Medicine, London, Heinemann, 1964.
9. Milani-Camparetti, A.: Spasticity versus patterned postural and motor behavior of spastics. *Excerpta Med. Int. Congr. Ser.* 107. IV International Congress of Physical Medicine. Paris, 1964.
10. Sherrington, C.: The Integrative Action of the Nervous System. New Haven, Yale University Press, 1961.
11. Clarke, E., and O'Malley, C.: The Human Brain and Spinal Cord. Berkeley, University of California Press, 1968.
12. Saint-Anne Dargassies, S.: Neurological Development in the Full Term and Premature Neonate. New York, Excerpta Medica, 1977.
13. Bobath, B., and Bobath, K.: Motor Development in Different Types of Cerebral Palsy. London, Heinemann, 1975.
14. Drillien, C.: Abnormal neurologic signs in the first year of life in low birth weight infants: Possible prognostic significance. *Dev. Med. Child Neurol.* 14:575, 1972.
15. Nellhaus, G.: Head circumference from birth to eighteen years. *Pediatrics* 41:106, 1968.
16. Rosenthal, R., Scherzer, A., and Cooper, W.: Unusual etiologies in congenital cerebral palsy. *Rev. Hosp. Spec. Surg.* 1:36, 1971.
17. Saint-Anne Dargassies, S.: Le nouveau-Né à terme. Aspect neurologique. *Biol. Neonate.* 4:174, 1962.
18. Thomas, A., Cheeni, Y., and Dargassies, S.: The Neurological Examination of the Infant. Little Club Clinics in Developmental Medicine. London, Heinemann, 1960.

19. Paine, R.: The early diagnosis of cerebral palsy. *R. I. Med. J.* 44:522, 1961.

20. Capute, A., Accardo, P., Vining, E., Rubenstein, J., and Harryman, S.: Primitive Reflex Profile. Baltimore, University Park Press, 1978.

21. Paine, R.: The evolution of infantile postural reflexes in the presence of chronic brain syndromes. *Dev. Med. Child. Neurol.* 6:345, 1964.

22. Hogan, G., and Milligan, J.: The plantar reflex of the newborn. *N. Engl. J. Med.* 285:502, 1971.

23. Paine, R., and Oppè, T.: Neurological Examination of Infants and Children. Little Club Clinics in Developmental Medicine. London, Heinemann, 1966, p. 187.

24. Frankenberg, W., Goldstein, A., and Camp, B.: The revised Denver Developmental Screening Test: its accuracy as screening instrument. *J. Pediatr.* 79:908, 1971.

25. Harris, D.: Children's Drawings as Measures of Intellectual Maturity. New York. Harcourt, Brace and World, 1963.

26. Capute, A., and Biehl, R.: Functional developmental evaluation: Prerequisite to habilitation. *Pediatr. Clin. North Am.* 20:3, 1973.

27. Silver, J.: Familial spastic paraplegia with amyotrophy of the hands. *Ann. Hum. Genet.* 30:69, 1966.

28. Molnar, G., and Gordon, S.: Cerebral palsy: predictive value of selected clinical signs for early prognostication of motor function. *Arch. Phys. Med. Rehabil.* 57:153, 1976.

29. Nyhan, W., Oliver, W., and Lesch, M.: A familial disorder of uric acid metabolism and central nervous system function. II *J. Pediatr.* 67:257, 1965.

30. Dubowitz, V.: The floppy infant: a practical approach to classification. *Dev. Med. Child Neurol.* 10:706, 1968.

31. Scherzer, A. L.: The Infant with Cerebral Palsy: An Approach to Identification, Management and Treatment. New York private printing, 1973.

3
Planning for the Abnormally Developing Child

CONSEQUENCES OF ABNORMAL NEUROLOGICAL DEVELOPMENT

Discordant Maturation

As we have seen, a nonprogressive deficit of the central nervous system may initially affect the brain stem and influence tone, and expression and integrity of primitive reflexes. Motor development and sensory response may equally be impaired. There is considerable variability in the expression of these deficits and uneven developmental growth is frequent. Thus children may respond well to the evnironment, including visual and auditory stimuli, with a social smile. Yet they might be extremely floppy with an exaggerated primitive reflex pattern. Variable maturational strengths and weaknesses are often a source of confusion in determining whether in fact the child is normal. The apparent discrepancy in response, movement, posture, and reflex behavior may, in fact, be the initial basis for a parent's concern.

The uneven nature of neurological maturation may become even more apparent with physical growth. Varying combinations of deficit may be encountered including floppy or exaggerated tone, immature posture, and abnormal reflexes. Often these characteristics will be present in association with emerging motor problems or asymmetry. Such children are a puzzle to parents. They have some strengths but seem unable to progress in the usual stages. Or perhaps they are seriously limited in all areas but from time to time seem to be making some progress—only to fall back and again be the cause for concern. This is the basis for initial anxiety, often the reason for referral, and generally at the root of tension that may greatly influence interfamily relationships.

The Influence of Abnormal Tone

Excessive floppiness or stiffness of the young child may often be the precipitating cause of concern by the family. A sense of abnormality is frequently conveyed intuitively when the child is somehow recognized to be too flexible and difficult to handle or too rigid to accommodate in the various usual postures.

Hypotonicity is associated with postural limpness and generally severe head lag. Often head, neck, and trunk control is also poor. Difficulties in handling and positioning the child are apparent early. This is initially seen in finding a comfortable, secure posture for feeding, whether by breast or bottle. There is excessive head lag and considerable support is generally necessary for the neck and turnk. This is true in a variety of postures including burping, dressing, bathing, and carrying the child. Floppy infants are immediately at a disadvantage also because they are greatly limited in their physical ability to maintain a secure posture in which to interact with the environment. This could be the start of a long unbroken period of deprivation of contact and stimulation that may add to existing deficits.

Hypertonicity may have similar effects on the child, contact with family, and the environment. It differs in that excessive stiffness is more likely to be viewed as obstinacy by the parent or may be considered causally related to irritability. The possibility of a behavioral factor and emotional stress could be thus introduced early to complicate the picture further. At times, the stiffness enables some degree of "standing" and may lead to the erroneous conclusion that makes the child appear excessively mature.

Often tone will change greatly as the infant develops. As indicated in Chapter 2, it is not infrequent for the hypotonic infant later to become a spastic child and for initial hypertonicity to appear ultimately as athetosis. Change in tone patterns adds further confusion to the daily problems in management. This is particularly true when the family is sensitive and responsive to adapting to the child.

Finally, there is often variable tone of the trunk and extremities. A hypotonic trunk may be associated with stiff upper extremities. Change in position may affect this relationship as well as postural reflexes. The effect is to present much perplexity and many frustrations to those who deal with the child on a daily basis.

Sensory Deficits and Function

The visually impaired infant may have a peripheral deficit such as cataract, congenital glaucoma, or other structural anomaly. The deficit may be central —within the optic tract or possibly involve the optic cortex. Both types of lesions may also be present. The effect of visual deprivation will be closely related to the complexity of involvement. An intact child with peripheral visual loss alone will obviously not respond to visual stimuli but will be affected by other sensory modalities. In this situation it may be more difficult to identify early that sight is impaired since the child may interact fairly well with the environment.

A central lesion affecting vision is more likely to be associated with other sensory or motor deficits which limit the child's interaction with or appreciation of the surroundings. The limited overall reaction of the child may call attention to developmental abnormality at a very early stage. While the infant may not see in either case, the presence of a peripheral lesion alone does not necessarily block other avenues for contact and learning.

Visual cues expected early in parenteral recognition are missed initially although a smile or verbal response to contact may occur. Within a fairly short time the lack of visual response in feeding confirms the underlying parental anxiety. If a central lesion is present, there are likely to be associated abnormalities of tone and reflex behavior as well, further affecting development. At times, it may be quite difficult to determine on observation alone whether visual loss exists, either because the child otherwise interacts well or is totally globally limited. Examination by electroretinography or visually evoked eletroencephalography (EEG) may be indicated to ascertain retinal function [1].

Auditory loss is comparable in potentially restricting major environmental contact and the stimulation needed for early development. Extent of overall effect relates to the complexity of deficit—ranging from peripheral (conductive, sensorineuro) to generalized central lesions involving auditory pathways, tone, reflex behavior, and motor abnormalities. Often, hearing loss is not clinically recognized early, particularly if it is peripheral. It may also not be adequately considered in the globally involved child who interacts poorly. A variety of diagnostic procedures may be utilized to delineate the condition including galvanic skin techniques [2] and the auditory-evoked electroencephalogram [3].

Recent data on hearing loss and emotional and social development confirm a much wider effect than had previously been recognized [4]. This may be beyond the physical and developmental deprivation experienced as a result of limited environmental contact.

The effect, if any, of tactile, proprioceptive, and gustatory loss on the young developing child has yet to be fully identified. One may speculate that individually or in conjunction with a more complex central lesion, they each could contribute to further deprivation and raise the issue of an appropriate remedial approach. Perceptual deficits and cognitive loss as seen in the learning disabled and mentally retarded, respectively, are limiting factors which restrict the child's options for experience and learning. Those with the greatest deficit have the least resources to utilize other strengths for development. The more mildly involved, however, may be able to use other abilities effectively. Early identification of limitations in these areas is more difficult and the question of how to remediate effectively remains open.

Abnormal Reflex Behavior and Deprivation

To a greater extent perhaps than any other initial neurological deficit, abnormalities of primitive and postural reflexes may have the most limiting influence on development. The child who roots and sucks poorly will feed poorly. Indeed, a first indication of deficit may be expressed as "colic" and irritability associated with the feeding process related to poor sucking and swallowing, with air trapping and inadequate intake. A strong asymmetric tonic neck reflex will limit reaching out, having contact with textures, shapes, and objects in the environment. Rolling from supine will be delayed or difficult and progression to sitting, crawling, and ambulation will be greatly impeded. Similarly, persistence of the tonic labryinthine reflex, with associated trunkal extension, will delay and limit sitting. Crawling will be restricted by a persistent symmetric tonic neck reflex in which tone of head and upper extremities correspond so that extension of the head will result in extension of the upper limbs and obstruct movement.

Strongly active and continued primitive reflexes will also influence parents' ability to perform child-care activities. Marked influence is inevitable on positioning, holding, bathing, dressing, and feeding because of abnromal postures and associated easily elicited reflex responses. The implications for management as well as parent–child interaction are obvious and far-reaching. The continued active influence of these and other primitive reflexes serves to "trap" the child in an immature state and intrinsically limit possibilities for self-initiated contact with the environment. Thus, by virtue of the early neurologic deficit, the child suffers deprivation of experience and possibly social interaction as well. These problems exist in addition to frequent physical limitations to tone abnormalities and specific motor disorder.

For the slightly older child similar concerns relate to delayed or incomplete appearance of the postural reflexes. Late neck and body righting restricts rolling, sitting, and crawling. Limited or incomplete righting reactions affect trunk control, weight bearing, and walking. Here too, delayed expression of reflexes occurs in conjunction with other function-restricting neurological deficits which impair the ability to interact with and actively participate in the environment.

These deficits have an immediate and continuing impact on the child's ability to learn actively from the environment and participate in the process of socialization. Hence, the neurologically impaired child may remain passive, dependent, and out of active contact unless his or her specific developmental needs are recognized and an active stimulation process individually constructed. Implications for both education and socialization of the affected infant relate directly to the inherent restriction from the very beginning of development.

Specific Motor Abnormality:
Posture and Movement

The child with a focal motor lesion such as a hemiplegia may early show signs of asymmetry. This may be apparent in limited expression of Moro reflex or startle response. Paucity of movement on the affected side will be seen as the child is handled, positioned, and dealt with in all areas of child care. More subtle and generalized motor limitations may be present and will affect movement and limit progression toward the upright posture.

The presence of actual motor signs and restriction will be associated with deficits of tone and reflex behavior. Such a child may well be further limited in physically moving effectively in the environment. Deprivation of contact and the inability to participate actively in the surroundings presents a serious consequence that may further affect such a child's development.

Oral Development Deficits

Of the many parameters impinging on early maturation, oral development has perhaps the most far-reaching influence. Many dimensions must be considered and full details of evaluation are delineated in Chapter 5. The rapidly emerging literature in this field gives some indication of the extensive areas which must be considered [5–8]. From a functional point of view, the initial concerns relate to limited rooting and sucking reflexes with frequent concomitant inadequate swallowing mechanism. This is not unusual when associated with fixed central nervous system deficit. Inefficient feeding with poor intake and frequent air trapping often results and is accompanied by marked irritability and the infant's inability to be satisfied. This clinical picture is often confused with "colic" and may result in frequent formula changes or alterations in breast feeding. In fact, this pattern is often the first "soft sign" that neurological abnormality exists, and will call for changing the approach to handling, positioning, and managing the child.

As the child grows, the oral development problems may involve inability to chew and swallow solids, or to drink from a cup. Complicated multiple deficits in taste of the tongue and proprioception of tongue, lips, and jaw may all play a part. Limitations in head, neck, and trunk control may further limit maintenance of the upright posture in sitting which will affect the infant's ability to participate actively in the feeding process [9].

Abnormality in development of speech itself relates to hearing, intellibence, development of receptive and expressive language, integration of motor mechanism of the tongue, palate, lips, and associated musculature. Maturation of the breathing pattern from initially nasopharyngeal to predominantly abdominal in the young infant, to thoracic in the normally developing child, may also be impaired and affect the speech mechanism [10].

Thus a fixed central nervous system lesion may influence all areas of oral development through direct effect on the structures of the oral cavity itself as well as indirectly through abnormality of tone, reflexes, and motor behavior involving head and neck. The major consequence is again a restriction of normal active experience with the mouth, its relation to other parts of the body, and to the surrounding environment. As in other areas already discussed, the net effect is to place the child at an experiential disadvantage; to make him or her a passive participant; and to compel a role of dependency. In this sense the neurological lesion serves to entrap such children, to "fix" them at an immature stage where they may remain unless some active intervention process alters their relation to the environment.

DEVELOPING AN ASSESSMENT PROCEDURE OF FUNCTION AND DEFICIT

Determining the appropriate diagnosis and description of neurological deficits provides only one dimension in understanding the meaning of developmental disability. The functional consequences outlined above provide a perspective which must also be considered in achieving an accurate understanding of the child's needs and future requirements. As well as a systematic examination of the neurological and appropriate developmental signs, a thorough investigation of functional limitations must be made as a basis for determining the future course of action.

The starting point is a detailed evaluation of tone, reflex behavior, motor and sensory status, and posture conducted by the therapist upon referral following diagnosis. A procedure which we utilize will be outlined in detail in Chapters 4 to 6. In addition, a transdisciplinary team approach is essential to evaluate the sensory modalities such as vision and hearing, speech, social and emotional status, cognition, and the family situation [11].

For the neonate and young infant, especially, particular attention should be given to problems in management arising out of the deficits identified in the evaluations. For example, hypotonia will have obvious consequences for posture, movement, and motor development. It will also affect many aspects of daily care and management of the child with which the parent will require direct assistance and guidance. Implications for contact with the environment and learning must be given equal consideration.

Management evaluation should cover at least the following major areas:

1. Handling

2. Positioning

3. Daily care

4. Bathing

5. Dressing

6. Feeding

Handling the child refers to awareness of special requirements for carrying the child, for support, and supervision necessitated by abnormalities of tone, reflex behavior, or motor limitations. Various postures may exaggerate abnormal tone or accentuate immature reflex patterns, for example. Others may enable the child to assume a more physiologic pattern yet be consistent with the tasks required of the parent, and need to be emphasized.

Positioning is similar but relates to specific adaptations that may be necessary in order to deal with the child. What is the best position given the specific limitations for cleaning, bathing, dressing, or feeding? The individual needs will determine how these can best be accomplished so as not to limit further nor tend further toward regression of the level of development.

Daily care includes all of the demands for infant management which are made more stringent when the child is developmentally delayed. Physical organization of equipment and space is a first consideration with special attention needed for adaptations of crib, high chair, layette, bathing equipment, etc. [12]. Where there are problems of positioning and handling, the parent must be adequately aware of steps which can be taken in preparation for care and of how the child can be helped to be a more secure participant.

Bathing is a good example of a daily activity requiring special handling and positioning for the infant. Without adequate preparation the child may be totally unstable for support and sitting in a wash basin or tub, which could lead to increase in tone and exaggeration of startle or other primitive reflexes. Moreover, under these circumstances, a potential opportunity for positive contact with the environment and learning could be totally lost. Instead, with stabilization of the child from behind, and emphasis on a midline position, a secure upright posture can be obtained with comfort and freedom of the arms and trunk, allowing the child to participate actively in what can be a productive learning and socializing experience.

Dressing, similarly, is an essential activity with many opportunities for interaction between parent and child, and with the environment. Problems of abnormal tone and pathologic reflex activity, for example, could totally influence the effect of this activity. Specific attention to details of abnormal function involving positioning, handling, and movement patterns as dressing is performed, will enable guidelines to be formulated to deal best with the dressing experience. As with other areas of management a guiding principle should be to assist the child to a secure position so that the youngster can observe and participate actively, if possible, in the entire process. This may mean achieving sufficient relaxation through flexion of hips and trunk to allow diapering of the hypertonic child; it may involve obtaining supported sitting with the child being guided from behind in putting on articles of clothing [13]. Functional evaluation must provide an insight into the child's specific deficits which have to be considered in working toward this goal.

Feeding is the child's most complex functional activity. It directly incorporates problems of tone, posture, motor abnormality, and reflex behavior with the head and oral mechanism. As with other areas of management, specific associated abnormalities must be identified as they relate to the feeding process. Here too, the goal is to afford a positive, active experience for the child, to enable ease of care, as well as maximize potential for learning and social development [14]. Specific management and treatment techniques concerned with feeding are reviewed in detail in Chapter 7.

Assessment findings concerning existing deficits, functional needs, and recommendations for continuing care should then be reviewed by the team. In deciding how best to approach the child, consideration must be given to family resources and capabilities, availability of facilities and staff, and a projection of short- and long-range needs.

REFERRAL FOR MANAGEMENT AND THERAPY

Overview of Therapy Methods

Definitive approaches to therapy for the young child with cerebral palsy have been evolving since the first works of Jennie Colby. The recent trend toward very early diagnosis and intervention has greatly shifted initial emphasis away from orthopedic surgery, and placed major priority on global remediation of the existing developmental deficits. The physical therapy modalities in current use reflect a continuum of approaches which have evolved over the past fifty years or more for some and more recently for others. Unequivocal superiority of a given method, including the most recently evolved, has yet to be fully established by adequate follow-up studies. However, the general relevance of early intervention physical therapy in effecting significant developmental change is becoming well-documented [15]. The following schools of therapy are among those which have had the greatest influence on treatment programs.

Crothers

While not a unique treatment procedure in itself, the approach of Crothers remains a basic guide to involving the patient in a meaningful program and is implicit in many of the current acceptable methods [16]. He stressed the need for active movement and stimulation activities to prevent contractures and encourage participation, even in the most severely involved children. He also counseled against overprotection, to enable the child to be more independent and active. Considered truisims today, these tenets offered a new and comprehensive approach which included the need for individualized assessment following which the child could be realistically directed to appropriate activities.

Phelps

This method used an orthopedic approach with conventional techniques from poliomyelitis treatment regimens. Therapy of individual muscles was stressed. Emphasis also was placed on training in gross movement patterns and inhibition of abnormal movements. Deep massage was employed for muscle stimulation. Auditory and kinesthetic activities were used, particularly a combination of rhymes and music together with desired movement patterns, to develop a conditioned reflex [17]. Once the association was established between a musical rhyme and movement, the child was expected to perform the movement upon hearing or reciting the rhyme.

Phelps encouraged visual stimulation with eye–hand coordination activities. Particular stress was placed on the use of orthotic devices for regulation of tone and postural adjustment. Relaxation techniques were used for dyskinesias; synergistic movement patterns were used, i.e., resisting one muscle group, to achieve movement in synergy. For example, he provided resistance to hip flexors in order to activate foot dorsiflexors.

Weights were highly regarded in treatment of ataxia. Stretching exercises were advocated for spasticity, with a heavy emphasis on the use of full control braces. The goal would be to reduce the extent of bracing as control was achieved about a particular joint.

In many respects, Phelps was the first to develop a coherent systematic approach. Much of his teaching remains in active use today in some form.

Deaver

His emphasis was on functional ability rather than patterns of movement, and objectives included [18]:

1. Performance of bed and wheelchair activities
2. Maximum use of hands
3. Performance of ambulation and stair climbing
4. Achievement of adequate speech and hearing
5. Achievement of as near normal appearance as possible

The method was to employ extensive bracing, restricting all but two movements of an extremity in functional activity. Reduction in extent of bracing would occur as functional control was achieved.

Considerable emphasis was placed on intensive training as well in activities of daily living (ADL), particularly wheel chair use [19]. For this purpose periods of treatment were prescribed in a residential unit, at frequent intervals as the child developed and needed to acquire new skills for function. Finally, surgery was often recommended for cosmetic reasons alone, such as to improve wrist flexion, or provide ankle stabilization, even when functional change would not be expected.

Fay-Doman

Fay, a neurophysiologist, early postulated the concept of motor developmental levels of the brain comparable to the evolutionary process [20]. The most primitive levels relate to the lowest forms and development progresses through maturation at each level. Thus the brain must evolve through stages of fish, and reptile, for example, finally toward mammalian species and ultimately humans. This highly controversial concept is frequently expressed as "ontogeny recapitulates phylogeny," or development of the individual recapitulates evolution of the species [21]. An insult or injury to the central nervous system interrupts this process with fixation at a given lower or immature stage. Thus, the child with anoxia is fixed at a primitive stage from which he or she cannot appropriately evolve as homo sapiens without an induced process which mirrors the suggested evolutionary brain process.

Doman, a trained physical therapist, took these concepts and integrated them into a system of therapy commonly referred to as "patterning," In this system the child must become proficient at each level before going on to the next [22]. The child is placed in prone position, using various ipsilateral and contralateral patterns of head turning and arm and leg movements. Graded developmental stages are used progressively including crawling, creeping, and walking with cross patterns.

Ancillary stimulatory procedures may be used simultaneously such as inhalation of carbon dioxide and use of deep pain with pin pricks. Fluid restriction was also suggested to reduce pressure of cerebrospinal fluid [23].

The patterning procedure is practiced on a regular daily schedule, usually using four or more volunteers for each administration. Parents are intimately involved in organizing and following the treatment process and meet with professionals at regular intervals for assessment of progress and assignment of a new treatment schedule.

Rood

Equal emphasis is placed upon both sensory and motor aspects of movement in this system. The basis lies in activating muscles through sensory receptors, and then using a sequence of developmental patterns of movement [24]. The emphasis is on developing an early awareness of normal patterns since it is obviously more difficult to correct abnormal patterns later.

Sensory receptor stimulation is accomplished by using heat or cold accompanied by stroking or brushing selected areas along a muscle group. Heat is particularly used for relaxation. Selection of stroking or brushing would depend upon the muscle groups involved, degree of tension, or restriction, and response to stimulation. Developmental patterns of movement are then encouraged to achieve physiological function with reinforcement.

Kabat–Knott

The procedures utilize facilitation mechanisms to increase voluntary muscle contraction through central excitation. Exercises use large movement patterns to activate and strengthen weak muscles. Mass movements are also used to simulate normal functional activities. A variety of spiral and diagonal movements are also part of this "proprioceptive neuromuscular facilitation" which generally requires a cooperative and well-motiviated patient [25].

Bobath and Neurodevelopmental Therapy (NDT)

The Bobaths have had the most recent and perhaps most extensive influence in the therapy field. Their treatment system is a neurodevelopmental approach to the total underlying deficts that relate to tone, movement, and posture. The basic abnormality is impairment of primitive and postural reflexes and abnormality of reflexes is associated with abnormal tone. By extension there will be developmental deficits of posture, movement, and progression in motor maturation [26].

The approach is to evaluate thoroughly the state of reflex development, and its effect on tone, posture, and movement. Treatment centers around inhibition of abnormal reflexes to alter tone, and facilitation procedures of

reflex behavior to develop normal patterns of posture and movement [27].
The system has been subject to changes in emphasis and direction and continues to be flexible in its approach to understanding the total underlying neurological maturation mechanism.

The wide appeal of Bobath NDT therapy has led to extensive training programs for therapists throughout Europe and the United States. Certification
as neurodevelopmentally trained (NDT) has gained considerable status as a
mark of professional expertise in this field and is sometimes implied to be the
only recognized professional training for those working with children.

Recently, the entire concept of abnormal reflex behavior has been questioned by Milani-Comparetti [28]. He shows that increasing evidence from
intrauterine studies suggest reflexes are operative long before birth and continue to be present on a lifetime continuum. He suggests that stimulation
and eliciting of "reflexes" leads to a response which is neither normal nor abnormal, but appropriate for that individual. He further questions a therapy
approach based on "abnormal" reflexes. Whether this criticism can alter or
influence the treatment approach remains to be determined.

Others

In the clinical treatment situation many knowledgeable therapists use an ec-
lectic approach. They first thoroughly evaluate the total patient (deficits and
needs), both for management and stimulating treatment. They then choose a
variety of modalities from several of the established schools of therapy as the
basis of treatment. This selective approach offers great flexibility and gives
the therapist an opportunity to tailor to the child's needs as well as the professional's capabilities and interests. No particular term is given to what is the
most frequently employed method. Its advantages are easily recognized. However, an obvious disadvantage relates to its lack of uniformity and systematiz-
ation which offers difficulty in evaluating and comparing results. This could
be overcome by more exact description and identification of the procedures
followed.

Therapy in Relation to Other Accepted Treatment Modalities

Treatment of cerebral palsy by definition must deal with the developmental
needs of a multiply handicapped child. The areas of disability go far beyond
motor development and maturation alone. Moreover, there are finite limitations to what can practically be expected of therapy programs as the child
grows and develops. Therapy can be offered as the earliest approach to treatment but is now among many available modalities which have been shown by
experience to be acceptable for the complex needs of the growing child [29].

How they are used and in what relationships remains a matter of judgement and clinical experience, as well as availability.

Medication

The use of drugs to alter the motor deficit of cerebral palsy and improve movement has a relatively recent and generally unsuccessful history. Their use with infants and young children has usually been limited to patients in at least the later preschool years. A variety of muscle relaxants have been tried with little benefit [30].

Dantrolene sodium also has generated conflicting claims of benefits and may be associated with serious liver dysfunction [31,32]. Its use in childhood cerebral palsy has not been demonstrated to be effective. However, in the stroke patient with a hemiplegia it has shown evidence of some functional effect [33].

Tranquilizers, such as chlordiazepoxide and diazepam, have been used with some effect in relief of increased tone and movement in the athetoid child [34]. In conjunction with an active therapy program, these are considered by some to be a useful and temporary adjunct in the total approach to the child [35]. As with all of the drugs used, none presently offers effective and sustained relief from motor, tone, and postural deficits by itself.

L-dopa has been used in the athetoid patient with some conflicting results [36,37]. Generally, some early response may be noted, but long-term effects are not seen [38] and side effects often cannot be tolerated.

With respect to the major associated handicaps, however, drugs do play a significant and often mandatory role. Anticonvulsants are essential in management of seizure disorders and must be continuously reevaluated. Where indiated, medication for attentional disorder and hyperactive behavior, especially in the older child, is required for the child to obtain maximum participation. Drug treatment for the severely emotionally disturbed child also has a place and may be a primary consideration before specific therapy for the cerebral palsy can take place.

Orthotic Devices and Equipment

A variety of functional aides are now available for therapy programs for the infant and very young child. The prone board, corner chair, feeding chair, other adaptive seating arrangements, sensory and motor stimulating toys, and specialized feeding equipment are a few of the many new innovations that both therapist and parent can use to deal with individual requirements. Such equipment is increasingly being devised with an awareness of its potential value in motor development and teaching. Considerably less emphasis is now being placed on use of standing tables and other rigid essentially passive structural and devices to contain the child.

Bracing in cerebral palsy has a long history and was often employed as the definitive modality. Its use as a treatment procedure in itself is now not accepted since experience has shown it to be restrictive, passive, and generally without active carry-over. In conjunction with orthopedic surgery, however, it has a well-established place to maintain correction obtained and as part of an active therapy program.

Use of braces together with a therapy program has both proponents and detractors. Bracing is generally discouraged for the infant and very young child with generalized cerebral palsy, with the emphasis on therapy to help achieve head control, sitting, and initial weight bearing. At that point in development, many clinicians would consider offering some form of brace for the lower extremities in the hope of overcoming deforming forces and stabilizing posture and gait. Therapy and bracing then need not be exclusive but may be mutually supplemental in helping achieve functional development.

The child with an obvious early hemiplegia might be considered a suitable candidate for short-leg bracing at a very young age to prevent contracture and enable earlier weight bearing. Again, there need not be conflict with a therapy program if functional goals are clear.

As the child develops toward weight bearing and ambulation, appropriate use and progression to walkers, crutches, and canes must be carefully considered. Wheelchairs are also becoming more functional and many types are now available offering better maneuverability and ease of handling, together with better control of the child. With active involvement in a therapy program there is less concern about dependency on introducing a wheelchair early, especially if it forms part of a functional treatment program.

Surgery

Surgical correction of any brain lesion associated with cerebral palsy in the infant would involve treatment of hydrocephalus, possible vascular anomalies, cysts, or benign tumors. Intractible seizures may respond to partial resection of brain tissue or even hemispherectomy in highly selective cases [39]. Obviously if any of these conditions are a serious consideration, appropriate identification and surgical management is mandatory and has priority over any other treatment considerations.

The procedure of chronic cerebellar stimulation utilizes an implanted electrical pacemaker to reduce tone, control extrinsic movement, and increase function primarily in adults with cerebral palsy [40]. Limited effectiveness over a prolonged period and possible significant placebo response [41] require careful evaluation. This procedure has not generally been used with infants. It remains an area of investigative neurophysiologic engineering which only requires further evaluation.

Orthopedic care and management have a major role in very early treatment of cerebral palsy. In conjunction with other medical specialists and therapy staff, the orthopedist provides guidance and direction in conservative approaches to limit or prevent abnormality and use of special equipment. As the child grows and maximum benefit is obtained from therapy, bracing, and other conservative measures, orthopedic surgical procedures should be considered to overcome residual deformity and improve function. The judgment of when and how extensively to operate is the key to proper orthopedic care. Early and continuous involvement with the child provides the best hope for the most realistic and appropriate surgical intervention.

Corrective eye surgery for strabismus should be performed as early as appropriate to prevent amblyopia. Repair of cleft lip and then palate is similarly essential in the very young child. Other types of corrective procedure may be necessary and could be planned in conjunction with the continuing therapy program.

Behavior Modification

A positive reward system to stimulate new or alter previous behavior has become increasingly popular as a psychological procedure and is referred to as "behavior modification" [42]. A specialized aspect, biofeedback, involves voluntary change affecting physiological parameters such as blood pressure or heart rate [43]. Data from the psychology literature confirm effectiveness of the technique for many discrete types of behaviors, especially for short time periods [44]. It has been utilized in the preschool child in gait training to overcome equinus [45], and in the infant to improve head control and sitting [46]. Planning the target behavior and developing the reward or reinforcement procedure requires a joint effort of therapist and psychologist. Sometimes the procedure can be used to condition the child to the therapy session itself to obtain better cooperation and participation. The technique may have much to offer in a broader way than is presently recognized and deserves wider application.

Social and Mental Health Services

A major advantage of working with the affected infant is that it provides the opportunity of becoming totally involved with the family. Often the child is identified only after a period of diagnostic confusion and a long search for the appropriate agency. Anxiety and guilt are frequently felt by the family. Conflicting information and advice about care or treatment may be overwhelming. Physical problems concerning finances and transportation may prevent needed participation. These and other problems require an active social service program with involvement in the home when needed. Counseling and definitive psychiatric referral and care must also be available. Parental discussion groups in conjunction with the therapy program can offer the support and direction to assure carry-over at home and an atmosphere conducive to growth. Professionals should not lose sight of the fact that appropriate support and care at home is the major ingredient reported by older patients, in long term follow-up studies, to have influenced their functioning and development [47].

Special Education

Early intervention programs for cerebral palsy and other developmental disabilities are proliferating within the United States and throughout the Western world. The models vary considerably; some are home-based and totally individualized, others utilize group methods with therapists and educational specialists. These offer the earliest form of special education for the child and a new form of special education for the parent. Whenever possible, the therapy program should be integrated into such a total educational effort enabling contact with other infants and families. This can greatly influence early learning and social maturity of the child, and provide the support and direction needed by families.

Controversial Treatments

Management and treatment programs clearly require use of various modalities. Timing, emphasis, and application will vary with the strengths and orientation of professionals, and as a result programs will differ. This is a natural consequence of continual change in technology, experience, and results of outcome.

Some procedures are in use and may have appeal yet are strongly questioned because of methods employed or outcomes claimed. This is true for patterning therapy (48–49) and the neurosurgical procedure of chronic cerebellar stimulation. Hypnosis has been used with older children [50], and acupuncture has also been advocated without any evidence of meaningful benefit [51]. Optometric exercises are widely prescribed for perceptual motor deficits, coordination, and balance, but long-term effects are difficult to evaluate [52]. Diet therapy is commonly employed for behavioral and perceptual problems, including the Feingold regime and use of megatitamins. The former area in particular is now being closely scrutinized for possible relevance [53,54].

A field dealing with chronic disability always requires the search for new and better ways of approach. It is hoped that a basic principle of objective evaluation and relevance to existing treatment will be kept in mind.

Developing the Prescription for Evaluation and Therapy

Identification of the child with significant developmental delay or with a definite diagnosis of cerebral palsy should lead to referral for appropriate care without delay. The physician and other professionals should be familiar with relevant resources within the community which can provide needed services, or at least be able to refer the patient to a source of information. The present evidence supporting early evaluation and intervention will be helpful in obtaining parental understanding and acceptance. Professional direction in finding the appropriate resource can help avoid "shopping" among agencies, ensure good communication, and avoid unnecessary delay in treatment. It is also essential that, following referral, the physician maintain active contact with the treatment agency to enable close follow-up of the patient and guidance for the family.

The referral for therapy is essentially a prescription and should include the basis for concern, diagnosis, and need for further work-up, and specific functional evaluation. These requests should first consider management problems to assist the family with care of the child. A full examination of sensory and motor development would then be expected so that the child can be placed in an appropriate treatment program. The elements of *management and treatment* should both be included in the prescription to ensure the most appropriate planning for the abnormally developing child.

Generally, the local medical society will have a listing of agencies offering services for the young child. State offices of United Cerebral Palsy can be contacted for location of local chapters where more information can be obtained. Easter Seal and similar other local agencies can provide information on relevant programs.

REFERENCES

1. Zapella, M.: The blink reflex to light in the newborn: Relation to light evoked cortical potentials in the EEG. *Dev. Med. Child. Neurol.* 9:207, 1967.
2. Vlach, V., Bermuth, H. von., and Prechtl, H.: State dependency of exteroceptive skin reflexes in newborn infants. *Dev. Med. Child Neurol.* 11:353, 1969.
3. Graziani, L., Weitzman, E., and Velasco, M.: Neurological maturation

and auditory evoked responses in low birth weight infants. *Pediatrics* 41:483, 1968.

4. Cavins, G., and Butterfield, E.: Assessing infant's auditory functioning. In Friedlander, B. et al. (Ed.): Exceptional Infant, Vol. III. New York, Brunner, Mazel, 1973, pp, 84–108.

5. Ingram, T.: Clinical significance of the infantile feeding reflexes. *Dev. Med. Child Neurol.* 4:159, 1962.

6. Logan, W., and Bosma, J.: Oral and pharyngeal disphagia in infancy. *Ped. Clin. North Am.* 14:47, 1967.

7. Brown, J.: Feeding reflexes in infancy. *Dev. Med. Child Neurol.* 11:641, 1969.

8. Bosma, F. (Ed.): Second Symposium on Oral Sensation and Perception. Springfield, Chas. C Thomas, 1970.

9. Adran, G., and Kemp, F.: Some important factors in the assessment of oropharyngeal function. *Dev. Med. Child Neurol.* 12:158, 1970.

10. Cook, C., Lucey, J., Drorbaugh, J., Segal, S., Sutherland, J., and Smith, C.: Apnea and respiratory distress in the newborn infant. *N. Engl. J. Med.* 254:562, 1956.

11. Haynes, U.: A Developmental Approach to Case Finding with Special Reference to Cerebral Palsy, Mental Retardation, and Mental Disorders. Washington, D.C., Public Health Service Publication No. 2017, 1970.

12. Finnie, N.: Handling the Young Cerebral Palsied Child at Home. New York, Dutton, 1975.

13. Connor, F.,Williamson, G., and Siepp, J. (Eds.): Program Guide for Infants and Toddlers with Neuromotor and Other Developmental Disabilities. New York, Teachers' College Press, 1978.

14. Sholl, C., and Scherzer, A.: Feeding problems of the cerebral palsied infant. *Pediatr. Dig.* 16:19, 1974.

15. Tjossem, T., (Ed.): Intervention Strategies for High Risk Infants and Young Children. Baltimore, University Park Press, 1976.

16. Crothers, B.: Disorders of the Nervous System in Childhood. New York, Appleton, 1926.

17. Phelps, W.: The rehabilitation of cerebral palsy. *South. Med. J.* 34:770, 1941.

18. Deaver, G.: Methods of treating the neuromuscular disabilities. *Arch. Phys. Med. Rehabil.* 37:363, 1956.

19. Deaver, G.: Cerebral Palsy: Methods of Evaluation and Treatment. Rehabilitation Monograph IX. New York, Institute for Rehabilitation Medicine, 1952.

20. Fay, T.: The use of pathological and unlocking reflexes in the rehabilitation of spastics. *Am. J. Phys. Med.* 33:347, 1954.

21. Gould, S.: Ontogeny and Phylogeny. Cambridge, Harvard University Press. 1977.

22. Doman, R., Spitz, E., Zucman, E., Delacato, C., and Doman, G.: Children with severe brain injuries. Neurological organization in terms of mobility. *JAMA* 174:257, 1960.

23. Gilette, H.: Systems of Therapy in Cerebral Palsy. Springfield, Chas. C Thomas, 1969.

24. Rood, M.: Neurophysiological mechanisms utilized in the treatment of neuromuscular dysfunction. *Am. J. Occup. Ther.* 10:4, 1956.

25. Knott, M., and Voss, D.: Proprioceptive Neuromuscular Facilitation, Patterns and Techniques. New York, Hoeber, 1963.

26. Bobath, K., and Bobath, B. The facilitation of normal postural reactions and movements in the treatment of cerebral palsy. *Physiotherapy* 50: 246, 1964.

27. Bobath, K., and Bobath, B.: Cerebral Palsy. In Pearson, P. (Ed.)., Physical Therapy in the Developmental Disabilities. Springfield, Chas. C Thomas, 1972, pp. 31–185.

28. Milani-Comparetti, A.: Fetal movements and cerebral palsy—a new classification. San Francisco, American Academy for Cerebral Palsy and Developmental Medicine, 1979.

29. Silver, L.: Acceptable and controversial approaches to treating the child with learning disabilities. *Pediatrics.* 55:406, 1975.

30. Denhoff, E.: Drugs in Cerebral Palsy. Clinics in Developmental Medicine. London, Heinemann, 1964.

31. Herman, R., Mayer, N., and Mecomber, S.: Clinical pharmaco-physiology of dantrolene sodium. *Am. J. Phys. Med.* 51:296, 1972.

32. Chyatte, S., Birdsong, J., and Roberson, D. Dantrolene sodium in athetoid cerebral palsy. *Arch. Phys. Med. Rehabil.* 54:365, 1973.

33. Mayer, N., Mecomber, S., and Herman, R.: Treatment of spacticity with dantrolene sodium. *Am. J. Phys. Med.* 52:18, 1973.

34. Keats, S., Morgese, A., and Nordlund, T.: The role of diazepam in the comprehensive treatment of cerebral palsied children. *Western Med.* 4: 22, 1963.

35. Denhoff, E.: Cerebral palsy—pharmacologic approach. *Clin. Pharmacol. Ther.* 5:947, 1964.

36. Rosenthal, R., McDowell, F., and Cooper, W.: Levodopa therapy in athetoid cerebral palsy: a preliminary report. *Neurology* 22:1, 1972.

37. Goodman, A., Goodman, L., and Gilman, A.: The Pharmacological Basis of Therapeutics. New York, MacMillan, 1980, p. 487.

38. McDowell, F., Lee, J., and Sweet, R.: Extrapyramidal Disease. In Baker, A., and Baker, L. (Eds): Clinical Neurology. New York, Harper and Row, 1978, vol. 2, p. 49.

39. Davidson, S., Falconer, M., and Stroud, C.: The place of surgery in the treatment of epilepsy in childhood and adolescence. *Dev. Med. Child Neurol.* 14:796, 1972.

40. Cooper, I., Riklan, M., Amin, I., Waltz, J., and Cullinan, T.: Chronic cerebellar stimulation in cerebral palsy. *Neurology* 26:744, 1976.
41. Medical News. Chronic cerebellar stimulation. *JAMA* 242:315, 1979.
42. Bandura, A.: Principles of Behavior Modification. New York, Holt, Rinehart and Winston, 1969.
43. Green, E., Green, A., and Walters, E.: Voluntary control of internal states: psychological and physiological. *J. Trans. Pers. Psychol.* 2:1, 1970.
44. Hawkins, R., Peterson, R., Schweid, E., and Bijou, S.: Behavior therapy in the home. Amelioration of problem parent-child relations with the parent in a therapeutic role. *J. Exp. Psychol.* 4:99, 1966.
45. Block, J., and Silverstein, L.: Integrating biofeedback-bioengineering approaches into a comprehensive cerebral palsy treatment center. New Orleans, American Congress of Rehabilitation Medicine, 1978.
46. Silverstein, L.: Biofeedback with young cerebral palsy children. In Feingold, B., and Bank, D. (Eds.): Developmental Disabilities of Early Childhood. Springfield, Chas. C Thomas, 1978, pp. 142–147.
47. Symposium: People with cerebral palsy talk for themselves. New York American Academy for Cerebral Palsy, 1971.
48. Freeman, R.: Controversy over "patterning" as a treatment of brain damage in children. *JAMA* 202:385, 1967.
49. Cohen, H., Birch, H., Taft, L.: Some considerations for evaluating the Doman-Delacato "patterning" method. *Pediatrics* 45:302, 1970.
50. Nieburgs, T., Goldenson, R., Nieburg, H., and Kline, M.: Hypnotic approaches to neuromuscular impairment: speech rehabilitation of the cerebral palsied: Atlanta, American Academy for Cerebral Palsy and Developmental Medicine, 1977.
51. Spears, C.: New approach to treatment of cerebral palsy: auricular therapy (acupuncture). Atlanta, American Academy for Cerebral Palsy and Developmental Medicine, 1977.
52. American Academy of Pediatrics. Joint organizational statement: The eye and learning disabilities. *Pediatrics* 49:454, 1972.
53. Conners, C., Goyette, C., Southwick, D., Lees, J., and Andrulonis, P.: Food additives and hyperkinesis: A controlled double-blind experiment. *Pediatrics* 58:154, 1976.
54. American Academy of Pediatrics, Committee on Nutrition. Megavitamin therapy for childhood psychoses and learning disabilities. *Pediatrics* 58:910, 1976.

4

Normal and Abnormal
Sensorimotor Development

OVERVIEW

The infant who is given a diagnosis of cerebral palsy by the pediatrician or neurologist is referred to physical, occupational, and speech therapy for further assessment and for treatment. With increased availability of early intervention programs however, referrals to therapy are made as early as possible and preferrably before subtle signs turn into marked symptoms upon which a positive diagnosis of central nervous system (CNS) dysfunction can be made.

At this point, the infant has undergone a developmental evaluation as described in Chapter 2. A more detailed qualitative assessment of sensorimotor functions is now in place. Thorough knowledge of normal and abnormal development is a prerequisite for such a detailed assessment.

A model for general principles of sensorimotor development is presented and applied to the course of normal as well as abnormal development. Implications of abnormal postural and oral development are discussed. Motor behavior is analyzed more specifically as to the underlying postural reflex mechanism and to intrinsic motor components which determine quality of postural alignment (function of righting reactions) and the degree of postural control (function of equilibrium reactions). Using illustrations, components of various abnormal movement patterns are contrasted with normal responses. The interaction between various movement components is described.

In abnormal development, important components of posture and movement are lacking. The baby is ill-prepared for subsequent developmental skills and more and more abnormal responses are perpetuated. Sensorimotor behavior, when seen in a truly developmental sense, can be interpreted as the summation of preceeding experiences as well as a preparation for future motor skills. Abnormal components of movement, even when subtle, can have alarming significance as potential obstacles to normal sensorimotor development.

GENERALIZED CONCEPTS OF SENSORIMOTOR DEVELOPMENT

NORMAL DEVELOPMENT

Research points to the presence of vast prenatal experiences in motor activity and sensation of movements. Fetal movements display an organization into clearly defined motor patterns [1,2], and the repertoire of postnatal movements and motor activities seems to be mostly a reflection and continuation of fetal motor patterns.

The neonate, although often described as functioning on a reflex level, is nevertheless equipped with a sizable variability of motor patterns. However, the postural control against gravity is very limited during the first weeks and months of life. The first year in particular, and to a substantial part the following four to five years are dedicated to the acquisition of this postural control and balance. The automatic responses mostly responsible for this control are the righting and equilibrium reactions.

The development of postural control proceeds generally in a cephalo to caudal direction as well as in a proximal to distal direction. The baby first acquires postural control and balance of the head before trunk balance and, finally, the ability to control movements of the pelvis and legs. Similarly, postural stability of the shoulder girdle, for example, prepares the development of skillful hand functions. However, the development of postural control should not be divided arbitrarily; and the interplay between cephalo to caudal and proximal to distal occurs in both directions. For example, head control can be refined only on the basis of some trunk control and shoulder girdle stability.

The child's acquisition of postural control and balance seems to follow a definite sequence relative to the three planes of the body.

Plane 1 Achieves control in the *sagital plane* with the use of extension as well as flexion against gravity.

Plane 2 Learns to the right in the *frontal plane,* using lateral flexion.

Plane 3 Postural control in the *transverse plane* is mastered through rotation within body axis.

There is, of course, a smooth and overlapping transition between these stages.

This sequence is repeated at different positional levels, i.e., in prone and supine, in sitting, crawling, and, finally, in standing and walking. It is interesting to correlate this pattern to the sequential development of movement direction in visual skills, in eye–hand coordination, and in the percept–concept formation. There, the sequence generally progresses also from the vertical to the horizontal to the diagonal direction, as for example, in building with cubes or in drawing.

A general pattern can, furthermore, be observed in the development of postural control of extension against gravity before postural control of flexion against gravity. The initial pattern of extension allows the infant to move out of a pattern of physiological flexion. Extension is then modified and graded through the counterbalance of flexion. Again, this sequence occurs in the different positions.

The extremities move from a mostly flexed posture which is exhibited by the neonate towards extension and abduction before full extension and adduction is established. Rotation is, again, the last component the infant learns to grade.

During the course of development, a progression can be seen from total motor synergies to dissociated or differentiated motor patterns. Initially, any action encompasses the whole body. Gradually, the infant learns to move one part of the body independently from other body parts and, furthermore, starts to combine components of different motor patterns, i.e., patterns of flexion and extension. Although some isolated movements can already be seen in the neonate, these are random. A persistent and purposeful application of selective, isolated and fine-tuned motor acts requires a high degree of inhibitory control, i.e., inhibition of total and excessive movements, and develops in accordance with the progressive maturation of the brain.

ABNORMAL DEVELOPMENT

Abnormal sensorimotor development may start in utero and the subsequent postnatal development of some infants may be a continuation of abnormal fetal sensorimotor experiences.

Early abnormal development is frequently expressed in exaggerated reflex behavior with a simultaneous absence of variability and adaptability of responses. Some reflexes may also be suppressed and weak, as for example, some of the feeding reflexes. In contrast with normal development where primitive reflex behavior gradually decreases while righting and equilibrium reactions emerge, central nervous system (CNS) impairment is characterized by an increase of reflex activity while righting and equilibrium reactions fail to develop.

Most often, however, sensorimotor deficits are not detected during the very first weeks or months of life. The symptoms of clearly abnormal motor reactions appear later and especially when the baby attempts to assume more upright positions. Without intervention, the severity of the symptoms increases during the course of development, although the brain lesion itself is stable and not progressive in cerebral palsy. Emerging abnormal motor patterns can be seen as a combination of neurological and kinesiological factors.

Abnormal development also proceeds generally in a cephalo to caudal direction and, depending on the distribution of impairment, initial symptoms usually occur in the area of head control and trunk control, while posture and movements of the legs may still appear normal. Also, abnormal distal movement components usually follow and can be traced back to abnormal proximal movements.

Sequential development of postural control for the three planes of the body is often arrested at the initial phase. Patterns of extension and flexion dominate the motor behavior, while lateral righting is often delayed and rotation within the body axis is impaired.

Patterns of extension frequently predominate and are not graded by a flexor component. Without the counterbalance of flexion, the antigravity extension differs not only in quality and grading but also in distribution (see Motor Patterns at Different Developmental Stages and Postural Control in Prone). Postural control of flexion against gravity is often poorly developed.

The last postural component of the limbs which emerges in a spastic pattern is the rotation. This is comparable to the sequencing in normal development. The abnormal extensor pattern, for example, is expressed initially in pronounced extensor tonus followed by progressive adduction and finally by internal rotation.

CNS dysfunction is expressed as a lack of inhibitory control. As a result, differentiated and selective movements cannot be executed. Instead, total and synergic motor patterns continue to characterize the motor behavior.

MOTOR PATTERNS AT DIFFERENT DEVELOPMENTAL STAGES

To identify a delay in development, it is important to know sequencing and timing of developmental milestones. There exists a vast literature on normal development. A selection of publications on this topic is included in the bibliography. To identify abnormal sensorimotor development as seen in cerebral palsy, it is necessary to analyze motor patterns and movement components which make developmental milestones possible. The analysis of motor patterns described in this chapter is based mostly on clinical experience [3–7].

MOTOR PATTERNS OF HEAD CONTROL

NORMAL

Postural control against gravity develops with the influence of righting reactions which brings the head into proper position in space. Some degree of head control is first displayed in supported upright and in prone positions (Fig. 1a). Newborns are already able to extend the neck and to lift the head briefly to free the nasal pathways while lying prone. At approximately four months of age, this primitive form of extension is altered with the integration of a flexor component allowing the baby to tuck the chin in and main-

Figure 1a (Normal). In prone, early righting against gravity is achieved through extension of the head (atlanto-occipital joint) and the spine (cervical and upper thorasic) bringing the face to a forty-five degree angle towards the support (two months). (Photograph by Christine Nelson.)

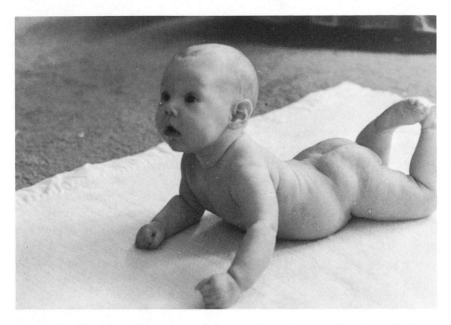

Figure 1b (Normal). More mature head righting indicates a fine interplay between extension and flexion. This brings the face into a vertical and the mouth into a horizontal position while elongating the neck. Free head movements can occur against a stable shoulder girdle (four months).

tain the face in a truly vertical plane. With the activation of pectorales muscles (flexor component), the infant pushes up on the elbows with more accent than before. The shoulders broaden and the neck elongates (Fig. 1b). Gradually, the baby learns to dissociate head movements from movements of shoulder girdle and trunk.

The ability to raise the head in supine comes somewhat later (by about five months). From then on the head is well-balanced in all positions. In upright positions the same posture appears as in prone. The combined activation of extension and flexion keeps the face in a vertical plane and elongates the neck.

ABNORMAL

Primitive posture. In abnormal development, the head posture is frequently affected. The primitive pattern of hyperextension of head and neck persists.

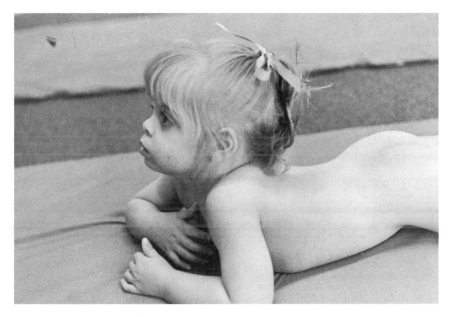

Figure 2 (Abnormal). Hypotonicity and poor coordination between flexion and extension lead this girl to raise her head with hyperextension of head and neck. Poor shoulder girdle stability interferes with free head movements. Compare with Fig. 1b.

Shoulder elevation usually accompanies this posture (Fig. 2). Head and shoulders move as one unit. This posture is basically seen in all positions.

Abnormal flexor tonus. In prone, abnormal flexor tonus may pull the infant into gravity. In this case the weight of the body rests on the head and the arms, similar to the newborn. As a result, raising of the head and the development of normal extensor patterns throughout the body are severely restricted (Fig. 3).

Abnormal extensor tonus and asymmetry. Any effort to move or to raise the head may result in extensor hypertonicity throughout the body. Predominant extensor patterns encourage asymmetry. Asymmetry of head posture may result in asymmetry throughout the body, especially when the influence of the asymmetrical tonic neck reflex (ATNR) is strong. Persistent reinforcement of this asymmetry interferes with the very important stage of symmetry and midline orientation. An asymmetrical head posture can also be seen in

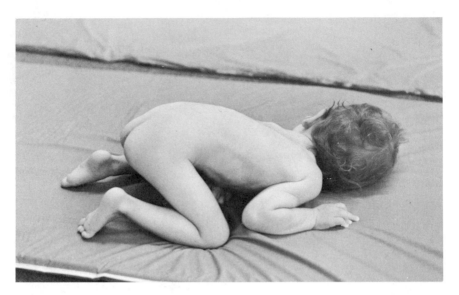

Figure 3 (Abnormal). Abnormal progravity flexor tonus causes this infant to weight bear on her head while in prone. Raising the head is therefore inhibited.

the hemiplegic child who orients himself or herself to the less impaired side. Rotation of the head is combined with lateral flexion to the skull side and with shoulder elevation.

POSTURAL CONTROL IN PRONE

NORMAL

Head lifting in prone starts a "chain reaction" of extension against gravity (Fig. 4). Complete antigravity extension is expressed in the Landau reaction which is obtained between five and eight months and which can be observed first in prone ("swimming" posture, prone on hands), and subsequently in ventral suspension. In the "swimming" posture, axial extension is combined and reinforced with scapular adduction and retraction in the shoulder joint. This motor pattern reappears later in the "high guard" posture in sitting, standing, and walking as a transient phase before some postural control and balance are developed. In the Landau reaction, neck and trunk extend and the legs assume a pattern of extension, slight abduction and external rotation of the hips, extension of the knees and, mostly, dorsiflexion of the

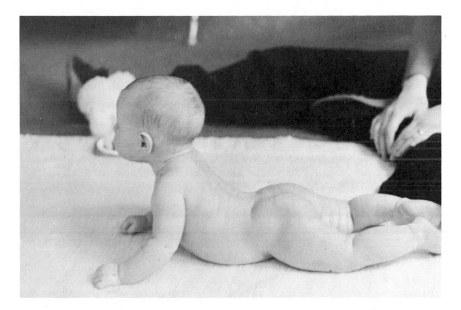

Figure 4 (Normal). The "chain reaction" of extension against gravity requires coordination between axial extensors and flexors (abdominals, extensors of spine and hips) in order to enable the infant to stabilize the pelvis and to raise head and chest off the support (five months).

ankles. A strong Landau reaction also provides the infant with some form of locomotion, for example, by propelling backwards on extended arms.

Complete antigravity extension can only develop when postural stability is allowed through the counterbalance of flexion. To raise head and chest off the support, the infant needs to stabilize the pelvis as a point to move against. Abdominal action and subsequent hip extension are required to stabilize the pelvis. Extension of the hips makes it possible to bring the legs closer together which facilitates weight shifting to one side. The weight shift promotes the amphibian reaction with dissociation of movements between the two sides of the body. This leads to controlled rolling, crawling, and creeping.

ABNORMAL

Abnormal postural tonus. Extension against gravity may be suppressed by abnormal flexor tonus which pulls the infant into gravity when in prone (see

Fig. 3). Very low postural tonus also restrains righting against gravity (Fig. 5). The effort to move against gravity may reinforce the development of extensor hypertonicity which is especially obvious in the posturing of the legs: adduction of the hips and plantar flexion of the ankles. Later on, internal rotation of the hips emerges. Although the legs are extended, the hips cannot fully extend due to the anterior pelvic tilt (Fig. 6). This pattern differs distinctly from the Landau reaction.

Poor integration between extension and flexion. When integration between flexion and extension is disturbed, proper righting against gravity cannot develop. In prone, the pelvis cannot be stabilized against the support and active hip extension is therefore not possible. As a result, weight bearing cannot shift down to the pelvis (Fig. 7).

Figure 5 (Abnormal). Hypotonicity is especially obvious in ventral suspension. Head righting and extension against gravity are lacking. Some hypertonicity is obvious in the pattern of adduction and internal rotation of the hips and plantarflexion of the feet. (From *The Infant with Cerebral Palsy: An Approach to Identification, Management and Treatment,* A. L. Scherzer. Private printing, New York, 1973.)

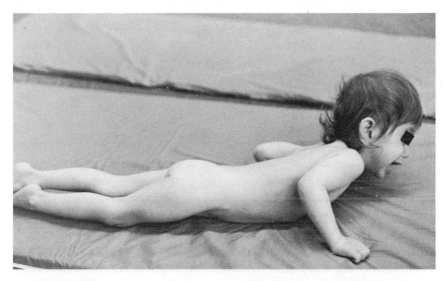

Figure 6 (Abnormal). Abnormal extensor tonus limits extension against gravity and results also in abnormal posturing of the limbs, such as adduction and internal rotation of the hips and extension of the shoulders. Compare with Fig. 4.

Figure 7 (Abnormal). When axial extension is not counterbalanced with flexion, the pelvis is pulled off the support and the body weight rests to a great part on the chest. The asymmetry of the head posture also indicates lack of flexor control.

Primitive flexor pattern of the legs.   A pronounced pattern of hip flexion and abduction ("frog posture") interferes with the chain reaction of extension against gravity. This also interferes with weight shift and locks the infant into a static posture.

POSTURAL CONTROL IN SUPINE

NORMAL

Although neonates display a flexed posture, they lack controlled flexion against gravity. During the first few months, extension activity increases, not only in prone but also in the supine position. The limbs which were initially positioned close to the body, move gradually into more extension and abduction. The increasing extensor tonus reinforces an asymmetrical posture which is highlighted in the ATNR attitude. This is most pronounced during the second month of life. A month later, active flexion against gravity permits the infant to keep and control the head in midline. Until then a sustained midline position of the head occurs predominantly during sucking and crying.

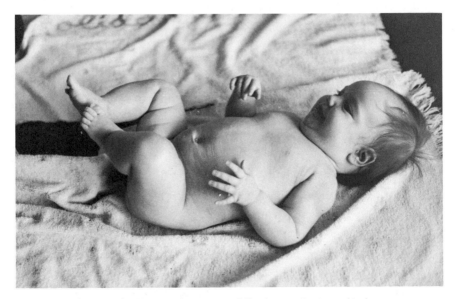

Figure 8a   (Normal). The development of flexion against gravity is necessary for sustained midline orientation of the head which produces a symmetrical posture throughout the body (three months).

Midline orientation of the head occasions postural symmetry throughout the body (Fig. 8a). The eyes start to converge, the hands come together, and bilateral movements of the limbs dominate.

Midline orientation and flexion against gravity permit investigation of the body. The eyes focus on the hands during play or while the baby reaches to his or her legs. With more flexion, the pelvis is raised off the support which brings the feet into the visual field and into the range of oral investigation. With a combination of flexion and extension patterns the infant raises the extremities with extended knees and elbows. While holding on to the legs the infant rocks from side to side, vigorously exercising the abdominal muscles during the performance of differentiated balance reactions (Fig. 8b).

Integration between flexion and extension can also be seen in the postural alignment of the spine. The whole spine rests on the support while the infant lies in supine. Integration between flexion and extension soon leads to new movement components such as lateral righting of the trunk, axial rotation

Figure 8b (Normal). Further flexor control enables the infant to elevate pelvis and legs high enough for the feet to be reached and to be in the visual field. Lateral weight shift and crossing of midline elicit balance reactions as a direct preparation for balancing in longleg sitting (five to six months).

Figure 9   (Normal). Initial attempts of rolling from supine to side are initiated mostly by pushing into extension. Nevertheless, posture of head and arms indicates control of both, extension and flexion (four months).

and differentiated movements of the limbs. All these new movement components enable the infant to move out of the supine position (Fig. 9).

ABNORMAL

Postural asymmetry.   Postural asymmetry persists when flexion against gravity does not develop. This is especially pronounced in the ATNR posture and causes lateral curvature of the spine and torsion of pelvis and trunk, especially when the ATNR influence is predominantly to one side. Lateral hiking and forward rotation of the pelvis on the skull side lead in time to adduction and internal rotation of the hip which is then in danger of luxation (Fig. 10).

Hypertonicity.   Extensor hypertonicity results in hyperlordosis of the cervical and lumbar spine. As a consequence, the pelvis is tilted anteriorly and the hips are in some degree of flexion. Arms and shoulder girdle are retracted (Fig. 11). Excessive flexor tonus seems to be mostly a secondary problem.

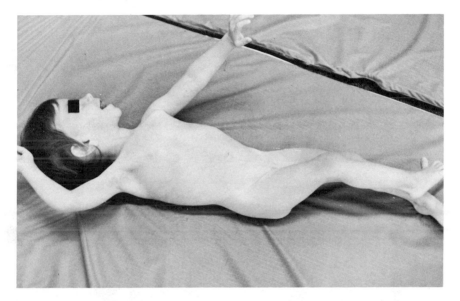

Figure 10 (Abnormal). A dominating influence of tonic reflexes (ATNR) pulls the right arm and shoulder back when the head is turned towards the left. As a consequence, this girl is unable to move out of supine. The pelvis rotates in the same direction as the head. Adduction and internal rotation of the right hip is a further component of this associated pattern. Compare with Fig. 9.

Lack of antigravity tonus. Flexion against gravity develops poorly when hypotonicity prevails. These babies usually assume a flexed and widely abducted posture of the limbs. The broad bilateral abduction interferes with weight shifting and does not permit a change of position. While these infants initially sink into gravity, they may, later on, develop extensor hypertonicity.

With lack of sustained antigravity tonus, body investigation and bilateral hand play are severely hampered. The hypotonic infant who is able to raise the feet off the support does so with marked abduction and flexion of the hips. Without abdominal action the pelvis is not lifted and legs and feet are not brought into the visual field. Control of the extremities in space is not practiced.

Some infants learn to use extension for bridging and even for some form of progression. In contrast with the normal pattern the extension occurs exclusively in the spine without any active participation of the hip extensors.

Figure 11 (Abnormal). Turning of the head, retraction of shoulders and arms as well as the wide abduction of the hips ("frog" posture) indicate lack of flexor control and suggest extensor hypertonicity. Compare configuration of chest and abdomen with Fig. 8a. (Photograph by Christine Nelson.)

Pushing into extension is also used for rolling and can, of course, not provide good movement control nor appropriate righting against gravity.

PATTERNS OF UPPER EXTREMITY WEIGHT BEARING

NORMAL

The newborn already bears weight on the arms when lying in prone. The majority of the body weight rests on chest and head and the ulnar side of the hand and arm. During the first month, the posture of the arms changes so that the weight bearing occurs on the palmar side of the hand (which is usually slightly fisted) and on the ventral side of the underarm. (The development of grasping starts also on the ulnar side of the hand, progressing to a palmar and, finally, to a radial grasp.) Gradually the arms move further away from the body into more abduction and the elbows are finally placed in vertical alignment with the shoulders (by about three months). This corrects the posture of scapular protraction and permits the development of independent head movements. With increasing balance between patterns of flexion and extension, the elbows move closer together into shoulder adduction allowing the infant to shift weight laterally when prone on forearms (by about four months) (Fig. 12a).

Increased extension activity of the upper trunk leads to increasing scapular adduction. Antigravity adduction of scapulae is most pronounced in the "swimming" posture which is exhibited in prone by about five months. Yet, in normal development, this strong extensor phase is offset by the forward-reaching in supine.

Dissociated movements between trunk, scapula, and humerus develop specifically during weight shifting in prone. These are important for the development of postural stability of the scapula and shoulder girdle preparing for more accurate reaching. Shoulder girdle stability also provides a stable base for controlled head movements. Lateral righting and movements of the trunk against the weight bearing arm are also practized in the side position (Fig. 12b,c).

In addition to weight bearing, visual and oral investigation of the hands as it occurs mostly in supine, prepare for the development of manipulative skills.

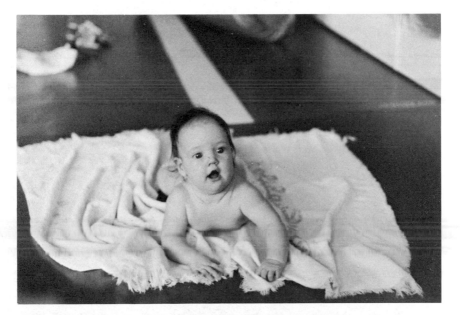

Figure 12a (Normal). Vertical alignment between shoulder and elbow enable the infant to develop balancing in prone on forearms and to maintain the alignment between head and shoulder girdle during lateral weight shift (three to four months).

Figure 12b (Normal). Lateral control is even more challenged in the side position. Lateral head righting elicits the amphibian reaction, which is elongation on the weight bearing and lateral flexion on the nonweight bearing side. The pattern of the right foot provides positional stability (six months).

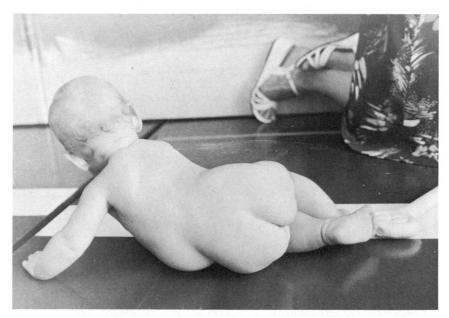

Figure 12c (Normal). Play activities in side propping require good shoulder girdle stability. Rotation within body axis is achieved by rotating the weight bearing shoulder back and/or by rotating the contralateral hip back (eight months).

When infants first reach towards objects, they overshoot their movements and require considerable practice in reaching objects accurately even when the hand is positioned out of visual field (five to six months).

ABNORMAL

Scapular protraction. In abnormally developing children, primitive patterns of weight bearing are often retained. In prone, extension of the shoulders causes the hands to be placed caudally in relation to the shoulders which encourages scapular protraction while restricting free head movements. Scapular protraction causes internal rotation and pronation of the arm, especially when combined with shoulder abduction. Internal rotation of the arms interferes with proper weight bearing on the hands. The weight rests mostly on the radial side of the hands. The hands are often fisted and may be positioned in ulnar wrist deviation. Strong internal rotation can result in weight bearing on the dorsum of the hand. Consistent scapular protraction interferes with the development of head and trunk balance. Intrinsic trunk movements such as rotation between shoulder girdle and pelvis cannot take place (Fig. 13).

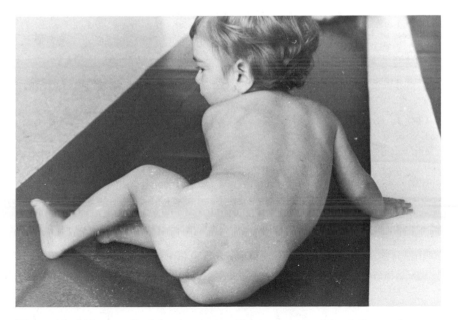

Figure 13 (Abnormal). Scapular protraction prevents axial rotation and makes balancing difficult. Compare with Fig. 12c.

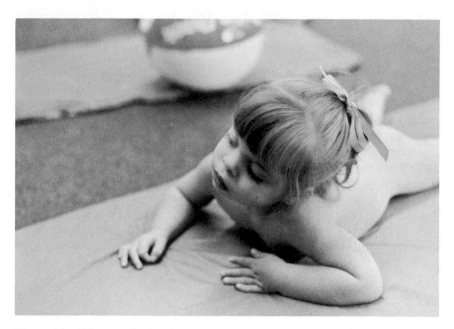

Figure 14 (Abnormal). A primitive pattern of wide shoulder abduction provides this girl with some postural stability but interferes with a balanced lateral weight shift. Instead of shifting the weight through the lower trunk and the pelvis, she tilts the head towards the weight bearing side. As a consequence, lateral righting is not elicited.

Lack of scapular stability. Coordination between patterns of extension and flexion is needed to stabilize the scapula on the trunk and to flex and adduct the shoulders for upper extremity weight bearing and weight shifting. Infants with poor reciprocal innervation compensate for lack of shoulder girdle stability with wide shoulder abduction. For lateral weight shift, the head is tilted which negates proper righting of head and trunk (Fig. 14).

Associated movements of scapula and humerus. Extension of the spine reinforces scapular retraction and shoulder extension. This "W" position of the arms is typical for the pure extensor pattern during early phases of abnormal development. The same posture appears at different stages of normal development and has been called "high guard." There it accompanies initial phases of independent sitting, standing, and walking before appropriate proximal control emerges. However, in a more stable position the normal infant moves out of the high guard posturing. In abnormal development this posture is maintained in all positions and the baby does not learn to move scapula and humerus independently, but continues to move them as one unit. In time, the mobility between scapula and humerus is drastically decreased and leads to excessive winging of the scapula whenever the arm is moved. Scapular stability cannot develop. Impaired shoulder girdle stability forms a poor base for head righting; also, accurate reaching and fine graded manipulative skills are impeded.

POSTURAL CONTROL IN SITTING

NORMAL
Infants sit square on their buttocks, with the pelvis perpendicular. However, due to lack of extension against gravity the babies demonstrate a rounded back in supported sitting up to about three months of age. From then on, extension progresses gradually in a cephalo to caudal direction (Fig. 15). When infants start briefly to sit unassisted, the lumbar spine may still be rounded (five to six months of age). To ensure balance, infants may prop themselves on the hands or may hold both arms in the "high guard" position. By that time, the infant has developed head balance but not full trunk balance in sitting. Head righting facilitates trunk righting (Fig. 16). Coordinated activation of extensors and flexors of trunk and hips must be achieved before equilibrium reactions emerge somewhat later in sitting [by about eight months (Fig. 17)]. Trunk movements can by then be better differentiated from movements of pelvis and legs. This permits, for example, flexion of hips combined with full extension of the lumbar spine. The improvement of trunk balance is expressed in a more narrow base of support, for example, the legs are no longer in a primitive and total flexor pattern but are brought closer together and extended at the knees. Secure sitting balance enables the infant to assume a variety of sitting postures. Furthermore, appropriate trunk control frees the hands for manipulation in sitting (Fig. 18). Preceeding and partially overlapping with the emergence of equilibrium is the development of protective extension of the arms (Fig. 19).

Balance in one position is only fully developed when the infant is able to assume the position or move out of it in a controlled fashion. During the early months of life the baby cannot effectively assist when pulled to a sitting position; and by four months is head control sufficiently developed so that

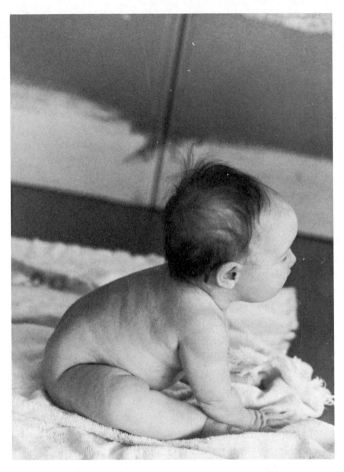

Figure 15 (Normal). Before extensor control of low back and hips develop fully, the infant leans forward in sitting. The legs are positioned in a total flexor pattern providing a broad base of support (three to four months).

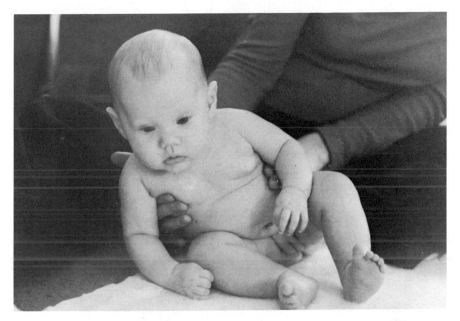

Figure 16 (Normal). When the center of gravity is displaced laterally, righting reactions ensure proper alignment of the head in space. The lateral flexion of the head elicits lateral flexion of the trunk and increased abduction of the limbs on the nonweight bearing side (five months).

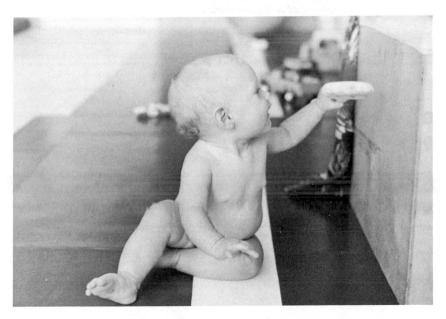

Figure 17 (Normal). Dissociation of movements between trunk, pelvis and hip allows a variety of balanced sitting postures (eight months).

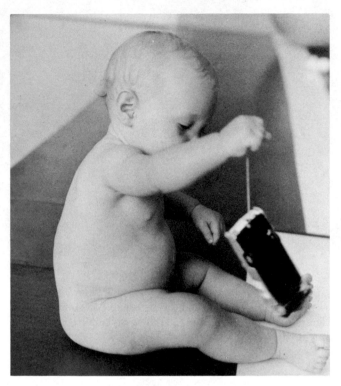

Figure 18 (Normal). Increased trunk control allows free manipulation of toys in supported longleg sitting. Control and mobility of pelvis and hips enable the infant to sit with pelvis and trunk in an upright position, to extend the knees and bring the legs close together (eight to ten months).

the infant can keep both the head and trunk in alignment when pulled to sitting (Fig. 20). With increased stability of shoulder girdle and trunk the five- to six-month-old infant can actively pull up when hands are held. Attempts to get to sitting independently are first successful from the prone position (seven months). Later, the infant rolls from supine to side lying and pushes up to sitting with the arms (ten months), while the symmetrical way of sitting up from supine is achieved much later (by five to six years).

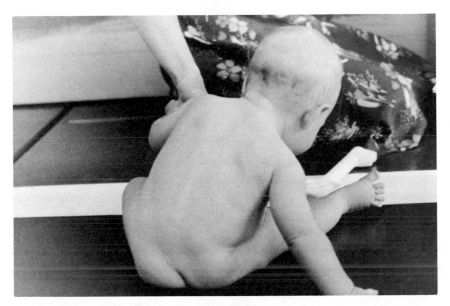

Figure 19 (Normal). When the center of gravity is displaced diagonally backwards, the infant reacts with trunk rotation and with protective extension of the arms backwards (ten to twelve months).

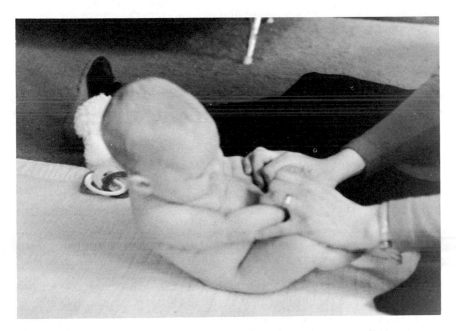

Figure 20 (Normal). Flexor control against gravity enables the infant to align head and trunk when pulled to sitting. Head flexion results in flexion throughout the body, including a total flexor pattern of the legs (five months).

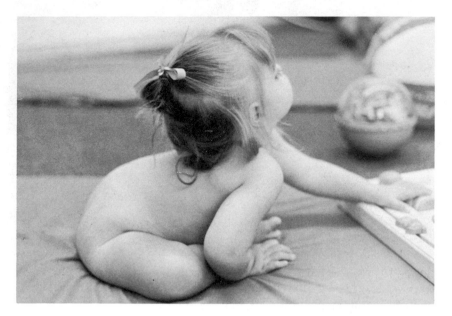

Figure 21 (Abnormal). Flexion of hips and lower trunk are excessive due to hypotonicity which causes this infant to collapse into gravity. Hyperextension of head and neck limit her visual interaction with the toy. Compare with Fig. 15.

ABNORMAL

Lack of extension against gravity. A flexed sitting posture, where the trunk falls forward into gravity, is typical for many hypotonic infants. The degree of flexion is exaggerated even in comparison with the normal neonate. At the same time, the head may "hang back" in hyperextension (Fig. 21).

Excessive extension. Some infants demonstrate premature and abnormal extension of the spine with a "high guard" posture of the arms. By leaning the trunk forward relative to the vertical line, these infants compensate for the lack of pelvic control. Wide abduction of hips provides positional stability and allows the pelvis to tilt forward (Fig. 22).

In other cases, abnormal extension may also be seen in the posture of the legs. Extensor hypertonicity leads to adduction at the hips and plantarflexion at the ankles. Later on, internal rotation of the hips emerges as a final component of the abnormal extensor patterns.

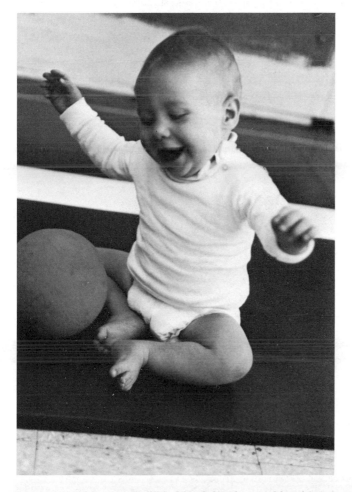

Figure 22 (Abnormal). Wide hip abduction enables this infant to maintain some stability in compensation for impaired control of trunk and pelvis. Compare with Fig. 18.

Compensatory flexion. The initial abnormal patterns demonstrated in prone and supine (see Postural Control in Prone; Postural Control in Supine) are often altered when the infant assumes a more upright position, such as sitting. Compensatory flexion of the upper trunk, neck, shoulder girdle, and arms may be superimposed on the total extensor pattern present in lower positions. Furthermore, head and mandible may be thrust forward. This occurs

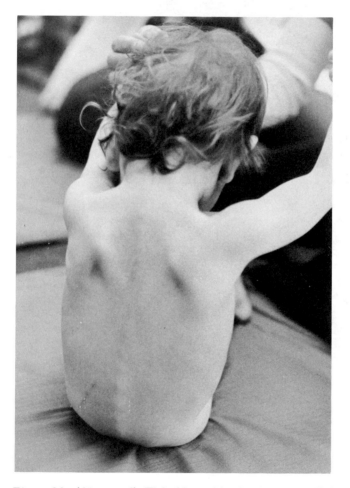

Figure 23 (Abnormal). Tight hip and back extensors pull the pelvis back to a degree where the infant sits on the sacrum. Poor coordination between extensors and flexors prevents an upright posture of pelvis and trunk. Compare with Fig. 18.

specifically when the extensors of the lower back and hips are shortened and, therefore, pull the pelvis back in longleg sitting. Contrary to normal, these infants sit on the sacrum (Fig. 23). Head, arms, and upper trunk are brought forward to gain some balance. For the infant to see the surroundings, the head must be tilted back. When the infant spends much time in this sitting posture, the compensatory flexion may increase flexor spasticity and may modify primary motor patterns in lower positions (Fig. 24).

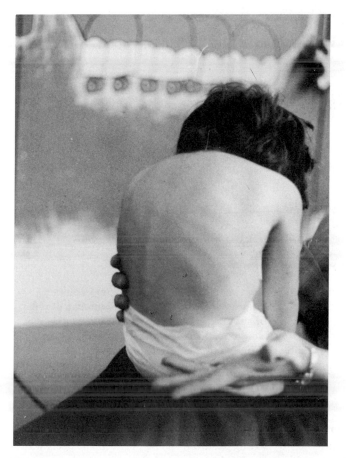

Figure 24 (Abnormal). Pronounced flexion of the upper trunk may develop as an attempt to counteract excessive hip extension and to bring the center of gravity forward over the base of support. Flexor spasticity may increase as a consequence which can lead to structural deformities.

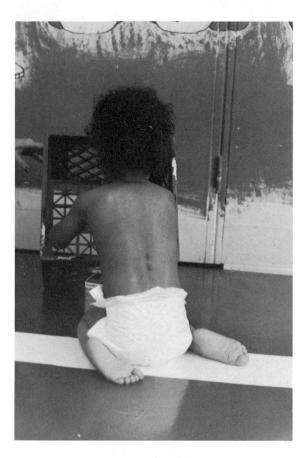

Figure 25 (Abnormal). Sitting between the heels ("W"-sitting) compen-
sates for lack of mobility and balance, and allows vertical alignment of pelvis and trunk. The broad base of support discourages any lateral or diagonal
weight shift resulting in a very static posture. Asymmetry of weight bearing
is common (see hips and feet). Consistent adduction and internal rotation
of the hips affect further development of the lower extremities.

    To compensate for lack of mobility and lack of balance the handicapped
infant often assumes the "W" sitting position: sitting between the heels which
provides a broad and stable base. This is a very static posture which does not
promote any weight shifting or the development of trunk and pelvic control
(Fig. 25).

Asymmetry of weight bearing. Predominant asymmetry of the pelvic posture is abnormal. It affects postural alignment throughout the body and patterns of weight bearing. Balance is threatened (Fig. 26). Some infants learn to sit unsupported by using head and upper trunk for balancing or by leaning on the hands but activities in such a position are very limited.

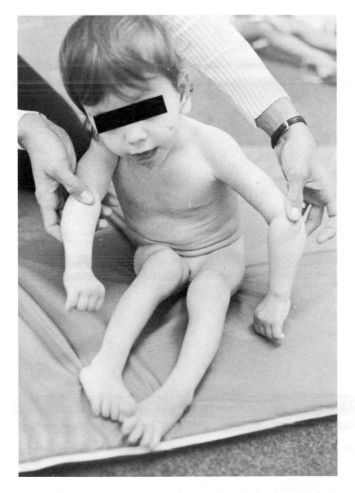

Figure 26 (Abnormal). Association of motor patterns results in retraction of trunk and pelvis. Alignment and balance are severely impaired.

Impaired righting and equilibrium reactions. In any of these sitting postures, the infant cannot develop good sitting balance. At best, the infant improves skills of compensatory patterns, but these compensations are restrictive to further development. As long as head righting is poorly developed, trunk righting cannot follow (Fig. 27). Due to poor head and trunk control the hands are not freed for manipulation, the shoulders are elevated with the

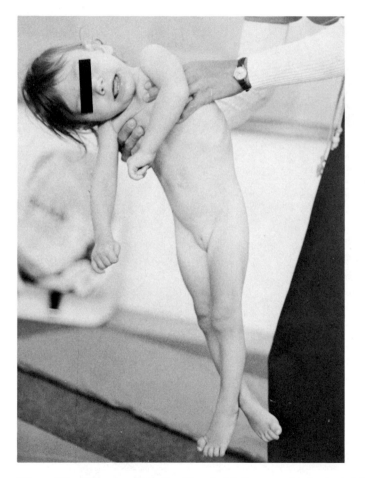

Figure 27 (Abnormal). Lateral head righting can also be tested in vertical suspension. With head and trunk falling into gravity, spatial orientation must be difficult. Compare with Fig. 16.

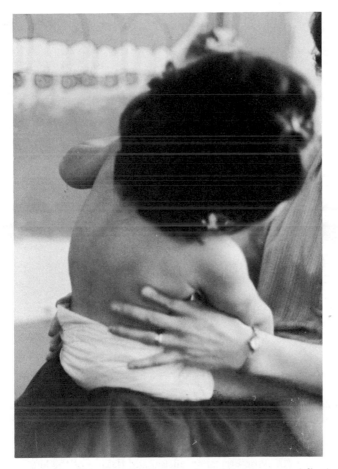

Figure 28 (Abnormal). Abnormal postural tonus and flexion of the upper trunk prevent this girl from rotating her right shoulder back for protective extension of the arm. Compare with Fig. 19.

scapula either protracted or retracted. All these abnormal compensations are a poor beginning for protective extension of the arms (Fig. 28).

Poor sitting balance is combined with an inability to sit unassisted or move into and out of sitting in a controlled fashion. When the infant is pulled into sitting, the head drops back and the shoulders elevate, indicating poor integration between axial extension and flexion (Fig. 29).

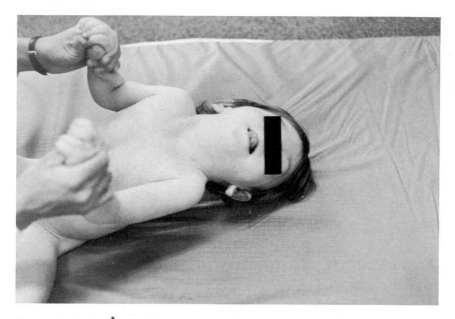

Figure 29 (Abnormal). This child shows severe head lag when pulled to sit. Hypertonicity is also expressed in the oral posture. Compare with Fig. 20.

PATTERNS OF LOCOMOTION

NORMAL

In the prone position, the neonate is capable of some locomotion in form of "crawling" movements, with symmetrical extension and flexion of the legs. The mature and more efficient pattern of belly crawling, however, differs substantially from this primary crawling and requires mor refined postural skills. Similar to any mature form of locomotion, crawling is initiated by a lateral weight shift. Before the infant attempts to crawl he or she has obtained much practice in lateral weight shift and lateral body righting, as for example, in prone on arms. The lateral righting of the trunk leads to a reaction of the leg, and the infant assumes the posture of the amphibian reaction: elongation and extension on the weight-bearing side, shortening and flexion on the non-weight-bearing side. By about five months, the lateral weight shift occurs more and more from the pelvis which causes the pelvis to rotate. This, in turn, permits the infant to pull the knee forward into flexion on the non-weight-bearing side. Now, the infant can push from the knee while both arms pull the body forward (at about five to six months). Gradually, the foot assists more in this action. First the infant pushes with the medial side of the foot; but soon he or she learns to use the toes to push off more efficiently.

With progressive differentiation of motor patterns, the infant is able to assume the fourpoint-kneeling position. Controlled weight shift is prepared for by rocking movements which, if vigorous enough, may result in the infant pushing the crib around. Initially, the stability in the quadruped position is ensured through a broad base. The hips are abducted and externally rotated. The back may sway slightly. Creeping in this position requires little active trunk balance. Trunk rotation is not yet possible in this position. Instead, the pelvis hikes laterally with each step. With the development of trunk rotation and equilibrium reactions in quadruped, the knees are brought closer together (under the body). By about nine to ten months reciprocal creeping patterns emerge. Variety of postures in fourpoint-crawling indicate increased balancing skills and differentiation (Figs. 30 and 31).

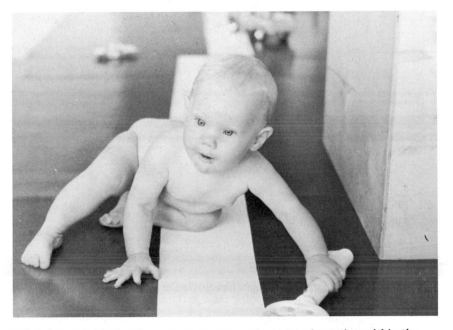

Figure 30 (Normal). Before the infant is able to control rotation within the body axis in the quadruped position, she rotates the leg under the body (flexion, abduction, and external rotation of the hip) while moving towards sitting. A high degree of mobility and dissociation is required for this maneuver (eight months).

Figure 31 (Normal). Weight bearing on the feet is prepared in many positions other than standing (see also Figs. 12b and 30). In this posture, the sensory input of weight bearing is reinforced by the infant's sitting on the heel. The right foot is in a state of readiness (push off) for a weight transfer or for a change of position (eight months).

ABNORMAL

The urge for locomotion may be strong in the handicapped infant but too often the child is ill-prepared for the task. Patterns of weight shifting are deficient even in less demanding situations as, for example, in prone on forearms. Head and body righting are incomplete. A tendency toward total motor patterns inhibits the development of differentiated movements such as the amphibian reaction or rotation of trunk and pelvis. Nevertheless, many handicapped infants learn to creep and to crawl, although in an abnormal and less efficient way.

Commando crawling. Due to their poor ability for weight shifting through the pelvis, infants may pull themselves forward exclusively with the arms while on their stomach. The effort involved causes, in time, an increase of extensor hypertonicity of the legs which are totally passive in this action. The legs are then extended although full hip extension is absent due to the anterior pelvic tilt and lumbar hyperlordosis. The hips are pulled more and more into adduction while the feet are plantarflexed (Fig. 32). This is a poor preparation for subsequent standing and walking.

While the weight shift in commando crawling is occasioned almost exclusively through head movements, some infants may learn to shift the weight more through the trunk but in an abnormal way. Using excessive extension, they wiggle and twist pelvis and legs from side to side while the legs are up in the air. The posture of the legs may simulate full hip extension but all the extension actually occurs in the low back.

Figure 32 (Abnormal). Commando crawling is a typical form of locomotion in abnormal development. Without lateral weight shift through the pelvis, the legs cannot actively participate and consequently the body is pulled forward with excessive flexion of the arms. The effort involved, increases extensor hypertonicity of the legs.

Asymmetry of weight bearing. The infant who uses mostly asymmetrical postures and movements learns to use both limbs (arm and leg) together in belly crawling, but only on one side. The head is turned to the same side and the contralateral side of the body is mostly ignored and "dragged along." In time, increased tightness of the nonactive side results due to associated reactions. Hypertonicity and tightness are expressed in the posture of the trunk (lateral flexion), pelvis (torsion), and extremities (flexion of arm, extension of leg).

Poor proximal stability. When postural control of shoulder girdle, trunk, and pelvis is poorly developed, infants compensate by shifting the center of gravity backwards over excessively flexed legs in the quadruped position (Fig. 33a,b). This interferes with lateral weight shift through lower trunk and pelvis. Important patterns of amphibian reaction and axial rotation cannot develop. Lack of dissociation of movements frequently leads to "bunny hopping."

The same abnormal posture of pelvis and legs is used in knee walking and affords a means of progression especially for the athetoid infant who lacks

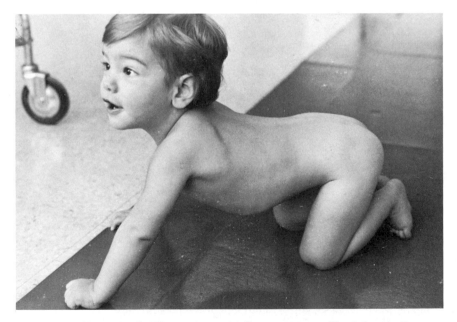

Figure 33a (Abnormal). The pronounced flexor pattern of both legs indicates poor proximal control. Lack of postural refinement leads to weight bearing on the dorsum of the toes. Compare with Fig. 31.

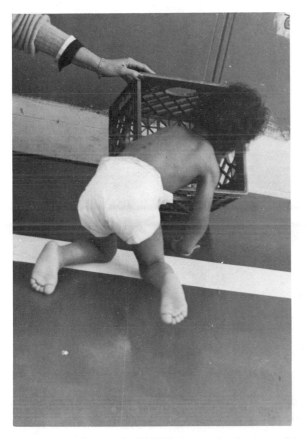

Figure 33b (Abnormal). With increasing hypertonicity the more primitive flexor pattern of the legs changes and the hips pull into adduction and internal rotation. In this position, movements are very restricted. The infant can either "bunny hop" or sit back between the heels (see Fig. 25).

functional upper extremity weight bearing. Again, the pelvis is "locked" in a pronounced anterior tilt which inhibits any intrinsic righting and balance re actions of the trunk. Therefore, a change of position can only occur into "W-sitting" which further reinforces a very similar static posture.

Progression in sitting. When strong postural asymmetry is present, fourpoint-creeping may be totally omitted. Instead, the infant may learn to propel while sitting by using arm and leg of the same side as the contralateral side is "dragged along" and ignored, as in belly crawling.

PATTERNS OF STANDING
(SUPPORTED, UNSUPPORTED)

NORMAL

The upright posture of standing and walking represents a final stage in the development of postural control against gravity. This process starts with neonates' instinctive drive to lift the head while prone.

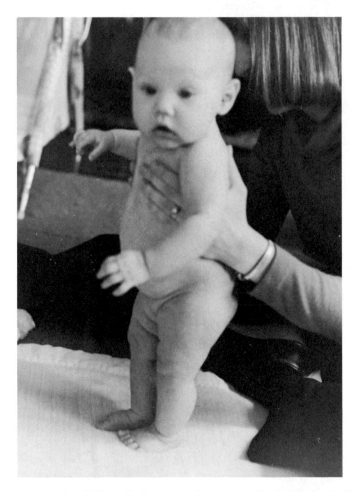

Figure 34a (Normal). During early phases of supported standing, the infant is unable to bring the hips forward for vertical alignment of feet, hips and shoulders. Weight bearing on the heels occurs with the knees in neutral extension.

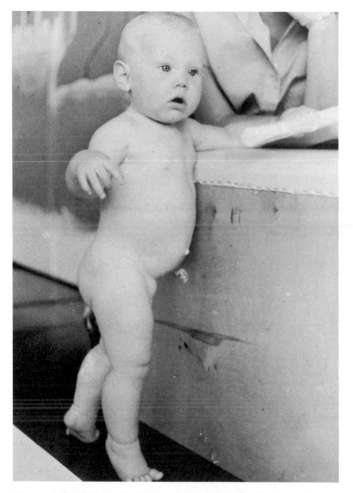

Figure 34b (Normal). While supporting herself, the infant moves between extended and flexed postures (toe standing and squatting). The center of gravity is now brought forward (eight months).

When held in an upright position, the neonate is already capable of supported standing and reflexive walking which are remnants of essential motor acts in utero. During the walking reflex of the full-term infant, the weight is on the whole sole of the foot, and the ankle is in slight dorsiflexion. This early skill soon disappears and emerges later in an altered version as a more controlled gait pattern. During early attempts at supported standing, the center of gravity is not fully aligned over the feet (Fig. 34a). Postural adaptations and movement patterns which infants have acquired in lower positions

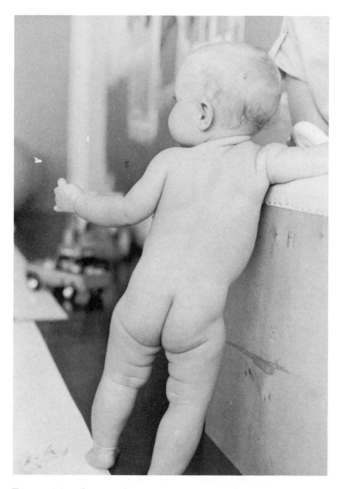

Figure 34c (Normal). Lateral weight shift and axial rotation are further skills which the infant practizes in supported standing before attempting to walk (eight to nine months).

are practized again in supported standing. Some of these patterns are: extension against gravity (toe standing and squatting), lateral weight shift, and axial rotation (Fig. 34b,c). Initial patterns of independent standing though, lack rotational components. Instead, infants assume a broad stance with both legs in abduction and external rotation. This is similar to the pattern of the Landau reaction. Their first steps take them along the crib in a lateral cruising pattern. The same broad base is maintained when they finally venture to walk independently. The first gait pattern is characterized by lateral flexion of the trunk and a primitive flexor pattern of the advancing leg. Since the infant does not apply pelvic rotation when walking, steps are very short. Hip extension and posterior pelvic tilt are not fully developed in this position and the pronounced extension of the trunk combined with the high guard position of the arms emerges, it seems, as compensation. The baby pulls to standing, moving quickly through a halfkneeling position when unable to maintain balance. Gradually, postural alignment and balance are more and more refined (Figs. 35 and 36).

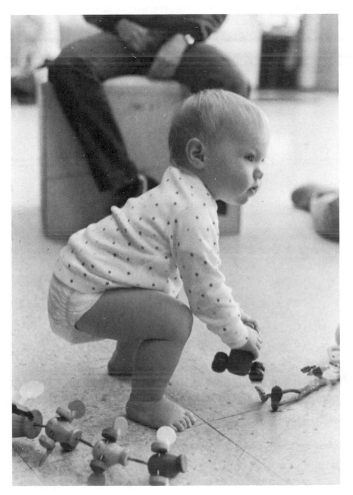

Figure 35 (Normal). A good sense of balance is expressed in the ability to squat without support (twelve to thirteen months).

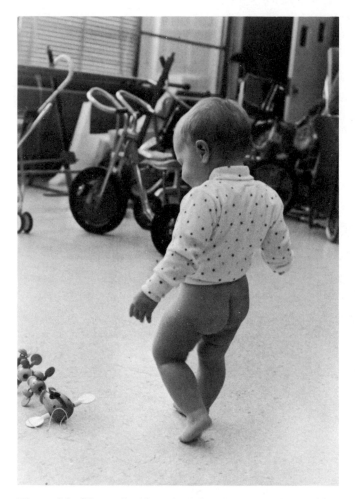

Figure 36 (Normal). After the infant has learned to walk independently, efforts to refine balance and posture must continue. Although this twelve months old infant no longer demonstrates the "high guard" posturing of the arms, scapular retraction indicates that rotation within the body axis is not yet fully mastered during walking.

ABNORMAL

Standing and walking are considerably delayed in abnormal development. Without appropriate intervention, the resulting gait pattern reflects most obviously the imbalance between different motor components.

Predominant hypertonicity.   Abnormal tonus affects the standing posture considerably and leads to poor postural alignment. Hypertonicity and the exaggerated positive supporting reaction cause plantarflexion, and weight bearing occurs exclusively on the ball of the foot. Flexion, adduction and internal rotation of hips facilitate pronation of forefoot and eversion of heel. This forms a very poor base of support and accentuates abnormal patterns throughout the body (Fig. 37). Without a component of flexion (abdominal

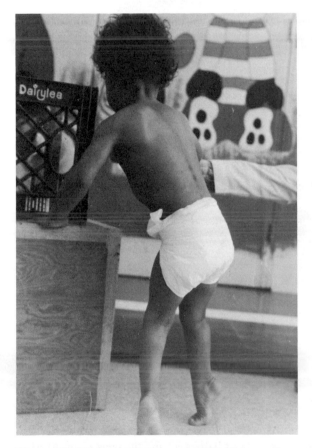

Figure 37 (Abnormal). Toe standing is frequently seen in abnormal development. Postural tonus, alignment and balance, however, contrast greatly with the adaptations of the normal baby. Compare with Fig. 34b.

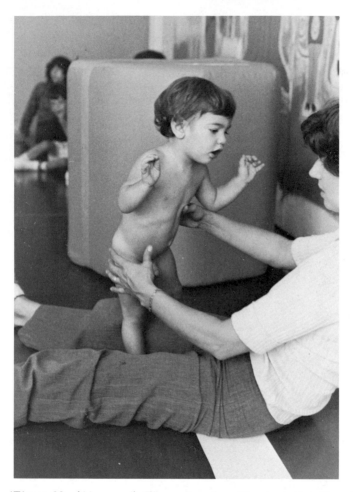

Figure 38 (Abnormal). The center of gravity cannot be aligned over the base of support without pelvic and hip control. This results in compensatory patterns of trunk, head and arms. Compare with Fig. 34a. (Photograph by Carol Herwig.)

control), the infant cannot align the center of gravity over the base of support and active hip extension cannot develop (Fig. 38). The infant with strong hypertonicity of the legs cannot half kneel and the great effort exerted to stand up increases the abnormal extensor pattern so that the child may bear weight on the dorsum of the feet.

Hypotonicity. The hypotonic infant may initially bear full weight only on the heel while curling the forefoot up in dorsiflexion and clawing the toes. In contrast with the hypertonic pattern, hypotonicity allows for wide abduction and exaggerated external rotation which shifts the weight also to the medial side of the foot and interferes with the development of proper balance reactions. The infant lacks active hip extension and pelvic control which affects postural alignment of trunk and head.

NORMAL AND ABNORMAL FEEDING PATTERNS

The vital behavior of successful feeding is insured from the onset through strong feeding reflexes: the rooting, suck–swallow, bite, and gag reflexes. They are already developed in the fetus and are active in utero. After birth, the different feeding reflexes must be coordinated with one more function: respiration. This coordination also seems to be prepared in utero where rhythmical expansions of the rib cage have been observed in combination with sucking motions [2]. A rhythmical interplay exists between sucking, swallowing, and breathing, determined by the sucking reflex [8]. From the beginning, the normal baby demonstrates some flexibility in this highly reflexive behavior and the capability to adjust to a variety of feeding situations. Infantile feeding reflexes become modified in the growing infant and, gradually, more mature feeding patterns emerge. For a more detailed description of feeding patterns see Chapter 6 (Observation of Feeding Patterns).

CNS impairment frequently causes disturbances of this highly coordinated and complex behavior and abnormal oral development is, thus, often detected at a very early age. When feeding reflexes are weak and difficult to elicit, tube feeding is often initiated. Choking and aspiration may result when coordination between the different feeding reflexes and breathing is disorganized and may be life-threatening. Adaptibility of feeding behavior is often poor, which restricts the infant to rigid feeding procedures and limited diets, often resulting in nutritional deficits. As with primitive postural reflexes, primitive and exaggerated feeding reflexes may persist, resulting in stereotyped feeding behavior which interferes with function as the child grows older. Feeding sessions may become unreasonably long while much food is lost due to uncoordinated and abnormal swallowing patterns.

Facial and oral motor functions cannot be separated from other behavior. Postural functions, such as head control, trunk control, and shoulder girdle stability have a strong effect on oral motor patterns. Graded jaw movements require some degree of postural stability of head, neck, and shoulder girdle. An abnormal degree and abnormal distribution of postural tonus may also be manifested in the oral and facial area, impeding fine coordinated and dissociated oral movements. Jaw thrusting, tongue thrusting, and retraction of lips and/or tongue accompany dominating tonic reflexes (Fig. 39). Predominant postural asymmetry or ATNR-posturing is also reflected in the oral posture and, if combined with abnormal tonus, may lead to subluxation or dislocation of the mandible.

Distorted reactions towards sensory stimuli, such as hypersensitivity towards touch and/or temperature, taste, and smell aggravate abnormal tonus.

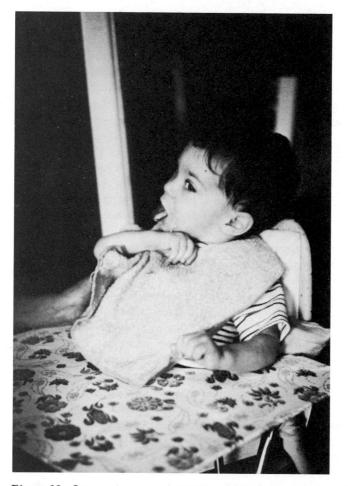

Figure 39   Jaw- and tongue-thrusting accompany tonic reflex behavior and are also an expression of exaggerated primitive feeding reflexes. (From *The Infant with Cerebral Palsy: An Approach to Identification, Management, and Treatment*, A. L. Scherzer. Private printing, New York, 1973.)

The infant may, as a result, give the appearance of total avoidance, adding even more frustration and tension to an already anxiety-filled and difficult feeding procedure. Positive interactions and communication between mother and infant as it normally emerges during feeding is curtailed. Instead of mealtimes being enjoyable and an opportunity for social interaction, they become a burden and a struggle for infant and caregiver.

Hypersensitivity toward sensory stimulation may also interfere with mouthing and thus deprive the infant of an important avenue of learning about properties of objects in preparation for future perceptual and cognitive development. The increasing refinement of feeding skills, as it occurs during normal development also prepares for other nonfeeding functions, such as articulation and speech. Primitive and abnormal feeding patterns delay or prevent normal sound and speech production. Abnormal swallowing patterns and abnormal posture of jaws, lips, and tongue result in excessive drooling. Abnormal oral function may impair dental health and contributes significantly to the development of oral and facial deformities, such as malocculsions and deformities of the palate.

REFERENCES

1. Hooker, D.: The Prenatal Origin of Behavior. New York, Hafner, 1969.
2. Milani-Comparetti, A., Janniruberto, A., Tajani, E.: Fetal Movements And Cerebral Palsy. Proceedings from Development of Movement in Infancy, pp. 1–37. Division of Physical Therapy, University of North Carolina, Chapel Hill, 1981.
3. Bly, L.: Normal and Abnormal Development. From lecture notes. Portland, Oregon, unpublished, 1978.
4. Bly, L.: The components of Normal and Abnormal Movements during the First Year of Life. Proceedings from Development of Movement in Infants, pp. 85–135. Division of Physical Therapy, University of North Carolina, Chapel Hill, N.C., 1981.
5. Bobath, B., and Bobath, K.: Motor Development in the Different Types of Cerebral Palsy. London, Heinemann, 1975.
6. Quinton, M. B.: Normal and Abnormal Development. Course in Neurodevelopmental Treatment. Unpublished lecture notes, Seattle, Washington, 1978.
7. Quinton, M. B.: Normal and Abnormal Development during the First Year of Life. NDT Baby Course. Unpublished lecture notes, Roosevelt, New York, 1981.
8. Peiper, A.: Cerebral Function in Infancy and Childhood. New York, Consultants Bureau, 1963.

BIBLIOGRAPHY

André-Thomas, and Autgaerden, S.: Locomotion From Pre- To Post-Natal Life. Clinics in Developmental Medicine, No. 24. London, The Spastics Society Medical Education and Information Unit in association with Heinemann, 1966.

Bèbe, M.: Mi Hijo Su Primer Ano. Buenos Aires, Sigmar, 1979.

Blankenstein, M. van., Welbergen, U. R., and Haas, J. H. de. Le Développement Du Nourrisson. Paris, Presses Universitaires, 1962.

Bobath, B., and Bobath, K.: Motor Development In The Different Types Of Cerebral Palsy. London, Heinemann, 1975.

Bower, T. G. R.: Development In Infancy. San Francisco, Freeman, 1974.

Brazelton, T. B.: Infants And Mothers, Differences In Development. New York, Dell, 1969.

Brazelton, T. B.: Toddlers And Parents, A Declaration Of Independence. New York, Delacorte, 1974.

Caplan, F., (ed.): The First Twelve Months Of Life, Your Baby's Growth Month by Month. New York, Grosset & Dunlap, 1973.

Caplan, F., and Caplan, T.: The Second Twelve Months Of Life, A Kaleidoscope Of Growth. New York, Grosset & Dunlap, 1979.

Casaer, P.: Postural Behavior In Newborn Infants. Philadelphia. Lippincott, 1979.

Gesell, A., Amatruda, C. S.: Developmental Diagnosis: Normal And Abnormal Child Development. New York, Hoeber, 1947.

Illingworth, R. S.: The Development Of The Infant And Young Child, Normal And Abnormal (3rd ed.). London, Livingstone, 1967.

Milani-Comparetti, A., Gidoni, E. A.: Pattern analysis of motor development and its disorders. *Dev. Med. Child Neurol.* 9:626–630, 1967.

Saint-Anne Dargassies, S.: Neurological Development In the Full-Term And Premature Neonate. Amsterdam, Elsevier, 1977.

Stern, F.: The reflex development of the infant. *Am. J. Occup. Ther.* 25: 155–158, 1971.

Touwen, B.: Neurological Development In Infancy. Clinics in Developmental Medicine No. 58. London, Heinemann, 1976.

White, B.: The First Three Years Of Life. Englewood Cliffs, N.J., Prentice-Hall, 1975.

5
Neurodevelopmental Assessment of Infants: Concepts

OVERVIEW

Symptoms resulting from damage to the maturing CNS vary considerably between individual patients. The picture presented by each patient also changes drastically during the course of development. The wide scope of abnormal development has been compared with the normal baby in Chapter 4. The assessment of cerebral palsy and related sensorimotor deficits cannot follow a routine approach but must be adapted to the individual patient. However, the underlying general concepts remain uniform for all patients.

A general orientation to assessment of infants is presented. Sensorimotor and adaptive behavior are analyzed from various points of reference. This allows grouping of the vast variety of reactions into few categories. In each category normal and abnormal behavior are contrasted with each other.

GENERAL ORIENTATION

Holistic Approach

The major focus of the therapist's assessment is the analysis of postural reactions and motor skills, including feeding. Postural evaluation must, however, go beyond the testing for various postural reflexes in an artificial testing situation. The therapist should instead observe how different postural reactions are coordinated with each other, how they are used spontaneously, and how they are adapted to different situations. Motor development cannot be separated from social, communicative, and intellectual skills. Furthermore, the evaluation process must be expanded to the infant/parent (family) unit. Sensory experiences and possible sensory restrictions must be considered.

Patterns of Posture and Movement

The major problem of the patient with cerebral palsy is not caused by a dysfunction of individual muscles or muscle groups but by a lack of coordination of muscle action. This is expressed in characteristic patterns of posture and movement, as well as in an imbalance between different motor patterns. The motor repertoire is restricted to few and stereotyped patterns, such as primitive reflex patterns while more mature postural reactions (righting, and equilibrium reactions) are impaired. Persistence of primitive and poorly integrated motor patterns necessitates more and more abnormal compensations as the motor tasks the infant attempts become more difficult. During early phases of development these abnormal motor patterns may alternate with more normal patterns. Identification of abnormal development based on disturbed patterns of posture and movements was introduced by Dr. Karel and Berta Bobath as a major concept of the neurodevelopmental treatment (NDT) approach.

Quality of Motor Patterns

The mere achievement of early developmental milestones does not seem a reliable sign of normal development. Instead, the quality of sensorimotor behavior relative to accompanying postures and intrinsic movement components must be considered. The quality of these automatic postural reactions depends largely on the quality of postural tonus.

Postural Tonus

Postural tonus is assessed on the basis of overall patterns and distribution throughout the body rather than performance of individual muscles. Posture and tonus observed distally and caudally are related to proximal patterns. Consideration is also given to the fact that degree and distribution of postural tonus can change drastically depending on various factors, i.e., degree of excitement, effort, orientation in space, postural alignment.

Automatic Postural Reactions

Functional activities, developmental motor skills and volitional motor acts
are performed on the basis of automatic postural reactions. Some of the most
important automatic postural reactions are righting and equilibrium reactions.
The development of these motor patterns is crucial for the development of
antigravity posture and efficient, controlled movement patterns. The interplay between different righting reactions provides a change of position and a
means of progression, such as rolling, creeping, etc. Equilibrium reactions provide postural control and balance. Motor components of righting and equilibrium reactions are integrated into volitional actions.

ADAPTIVE BEHAVIOR

Introduction

Immaturity and dysfunction of the central nervous system are frequently
expressed in general attitudes and responsiveness to environmental stimuli.
The quality of certain adaptive responses can therefore strengthen or weaken
the significance of suspect abnormal motor signs, specifically during early
phases of development.

Threshold for Stimulation

CNS dysfunction can be detected in the infant's tolerance to different stimuli. During the first weeks of life, normal babies display an ability to adapt to
a variety of stimuli and to organize themselves accordingly. They can adjust
to disturbing stimuli and, to some extent, protect themselves against over-
stimulation. Once aroused, babies find various ways of calming themselves.

The infant with CNS dysfunction may demonstrate an abnormally low
threshold to stimulation. This hypersensitivity can produce disorganized and
highly irritable behavior. Hypersensitivity may be revealed in the infant's reaction to auditory and visual stimuli and being touched. Conversely, the infant who is extremely "good" may be indicating lack of responsiveness and
abnormally high threshold to stimulation due to CNS impairment.

Variability of Behavior

Babies learn very early to modify their responses as well as to adapt to new
situations. Variability and unpredictability of responses, including patterns of
primitive reflexes, are important characteristics in normal development.

A very narrow repertoire of responses, and stereotyped behavior in areas of
sensorimotor, social, emotional, and mental functions, indicate abnormality.

Mental Responsiveness

Alertness and attentiveness are exhibited by the newborn although only for short periods at a time. The skill for selective attention to environmental stimuli starts to develop early and is very important for further mental development.

Lack of responsiveness may be displayed together with abnormal development. Pronounced distractability is another expression of CNS immaturity; it reduces the opportunity for early learning and may aggrevate developmental delay. Untiring repetition of stereotyped responses to the same stimulus contrasts equally with the typical response of normal babies. They quickly tire of too much repetition and seem to strive for a constant expansion into new experiences.

Social Interaction

Interest in the surroundings, curiosity, and clearly displayed pleasure in communication are characteristics of the healthy and normally developing infant. Babies make extreme efforts to achieve personal attention and seem to thrive on it.

Social interaction and responses to the environment may be suppressed and disturbed in infants with CNS impairment.

MOTOR SKILLS AND DEVELOPMENTAL MILESTONES

Motor output cannot be separated from sensory input. Movements are shaped by proprioceptive and tactile feedback and by visual, auditory, and labyrinthine orientation. A motor act is often prompted by visual or auditory stimuli. Quality and type of sensory experiences provided by the infant's environment must be considered as much as any sensory deficit.

A list of functional skills achieved by the infant as well as age-appropriate skills not obtained form one part of the assessment. Allocation of the infant's level of functioning to specific months and weeks, however, cannot reflect the true developmental deficiencies but can misrepresent the infant's true condition, especially when achievement of developmental skills is scattered.

The following outline organizes functional skills into major categories. The developmental level within each category must be adjusted to the child's chronological as well as developmental age.

Head and Trunk Control

The degree of head and trunk control which indicates the level of righting and balancing skills is evaluated when the infant is prone, supine, sitting, and while pulled to sitting from supine. Head and trunk control should also be evaluated in the frontal body plane, for example, when the weight is shifted to one side, requiring a lateral tilt of head and trunk to the opposite side and, later on, a component of rotation. This reaction can be elicited in prone, sitting, or vertical suspension. The infant with good head and trunk control is also tested for the Landau reaction: extension throughout the body with hips in extension-abduction and external rotation. This response is tested with the child in ventral suspension.

Upper Extremity Function

The skill in propping on arms or hands is observed in prone and in sitting. A test for protective extension of the arms in all directions is included when appropriate.

Hand functions, such as reach, grasp, and release are evaluated for voluntary control. Bilateral manipulation as well as the ability to transfer objects are skills to look for. A strong preference for one hand is suggestive of sensory or tonal asymmetries. Consistent fisting of the hands is abnormal. Hand play, body investigation, and mouthing are important stages of normal motor development.

Change of Positions

The ability to change positions is a significant motor function. Rolling from prone to supine and vice versa, moving from prone to crawling position, assuming a sitting position, and pulling to standing all give the baby some measure of independence. The degree of control and balance should be noted. Some infants may require minimal assistance to be successful in their attempts. In addition, infants should be evaluated in their ability to maintain a position they cannot yet assume unassisted.

Progression

Ability for and mode of progression are described next. A baby can move around by rolling, belly crawling, crawling on hands and knees or hands and feet, cruising, or walking. Some infants learn to progress in sitting, as, for example, the infant with hemiplegia who pulls himself or herself forward with one hand while 'dragging' the hemiplegic side along; the same retraction of the hemiplegic side may also be seen in walking. When assessing gait, the therapist prompts the child to walk in all directions, turn, and stand up with or without support. When asked to ascend or descend stairs, many infants regress to crawling.

Supported Standing

The nonambulatory infant is placed into a supported standing position to evaluate his or her capability for weight bearing. A test for the parachute reaction may emphasize abnormal posture and abnormal tonus. The parachute reaction is a protective extension of the lower limbs during sudden displacement of the erect trunk and emerges at four months (Milani-Comparetti). The legs assume a posture of extension and abduction and the feet are dorsiflexed. It is tested in vertical suspension.

QUALITY OF MOTOR PATTERNS

Introduction

Abnormal development is most obvious when age—appropriate motor skills are lacking and when developmental milestones are not reached. Early identification however, requires a more qualitative assessment including quality of postural tonus and quality of motor patterns. During the course of development, patterns of previously acquired skills are more and more refined, postural mechanisms become more complex, more sophisticated and, more efficient. Quality of movement patterns reflect the level of maturation and integrative function of the CNS. Well integrated sensorimotor behavior precedes development of numerous perceptual and cognitive skills. The quality of movements has, therefore, far-reaching impact on the child's future.

Knowledge of normal motor patterns and how they change in the course of development is an important tool for early identification of abnormal sensorimotor behavior. The most important normal and abnormal motor patterns are described in Chapter 4.

Postural Tonus

Postural tonus reflects the dynamic interplay between excitatory and inhibitory centers of the CNS and is receptive to exteroceptive and proprioceptive stimuli. Consequently, degree and distribution of postural tonus are changeable and can be influenced by the type and quality of sensory input.

NORMAL

Strength and distribution. Quality and distribution of postural tonus are expressed in patterns of posture and movements, and in the degree of ease or effort during movements. Normal postural tonus is sufficiently high to enable weight bearing and support against gravity. Yet at the same time normal postural tonus is low enough to allow quick and easy adaptations towards active and passive movements. A high degree of coordination between stability and motility is a prerequisite for selective, skillful activities.

Distribution of tonus changes during the course of development. During early phases, tonus is higher distally than proximally, and higher in the upper than in the lower extremities (Saint-Anne Dargassies, 1977). This pattern is completely reversed providing relatively more proximal stability and more distal motility.

Reciprocal innervation. Stability, motility, and the interplay between both is determined by reciprocal innervation which coordinates opposing muscle groups. With normal motor control a movement initiated by one muscle group (agonist) is guided by the gradual relaxation and elongation of the opposing muscle group (antagonist). When agonist and antagonist work with the same force, cocontraction occurs, resulting in either postural stabilization or proximal fixation.

ABNORMAL

CNS deficit causes an imbalance between centers of excitation and inhibition. Distribution of tonus differs from the norm and may reflect patterns of abnormal tonic reflex behavior. When distribution of tonus fails to undergo normal developmental changes, tonus remains high distally while it is low proximally. Balancing and manipulative skills are then impeded.

Poor support tonus, lack of righting against gravity, and restrictions of mobility may be expressed in the patient's spontaneous motor behavior. A more precise, qualitative assessment of tonus is achieved when the therapist handles the infant. Abnormal postural tonus is indicated in the child's inability to adapt to the therapist's handling.

Postural tonus may change drastically depending on the infant's position, activity, state of excitement, and amount of effort used. Therefore, tonus must be evaluated during different activities and in different situations, i.e., when the infant is at rest as well as when active and exposed to different stimuli.

Hypertonicity and spasticity. In the case of hypertonicity, the examiner feels undue resistance towards antigravity movements and undue assistance when moving with gravity. The degree of resistance may fluctuate throughout the range of a given movement. Strong resistance may suddenly disappear at a certain point (clasp knife phenomenon). Hypertonicity is also evidenced in associated reactions, for example, during commando crawling where the infant pulls forward with the arms which increases extensor hypertonicity of the legs. Clonus is another phenomenon associated with spasticity.

Hypotonicity. The hypotonic infant also lacks proper postural control against gravity. The limbs and body sink into gravity which is expressed, for example, in the typical posture of the limbs often referred to as "frog position." When moved passively, the limbs feel heavy because the infant cannot support their weight. Lacking resistance towards extreme movements, the hypotonic baby often displays hypermobility. Hypertonicity often can be provoked in the basically hypotonic infant with stress and brisk handling, for example, in a test for adductor hypertonicity.

Fluctuations of tonus and tremor.   Strong fluctuations of tonus can be felt in patients with athetosis. Involuntary movements, so typical for the athetoid patient, may be, to some degree, the result of these fluctuations. Tremor can often be observed in the ataxic child.

Disturbed reciprocal innervation.   Disturbances of interplay between agonist and antagonist vary. The spastic patient applies too much cocontraction, i.e., agonist and antagonist work with the same force. As a result, movements are restricted and require much effort. In the athetoid as well as in the ataxic patient a paucity of cocontraction contributes to a lack of postural stabilization. When the athetoid or ataxic patient initiates a movement, the antagonist relaxes too quickly and causes the movement to be uncontrolled and exaggerated.

Variability of Motor Responses

NORMAL
From the onset, the normal baby demonstrates a certain variability in motor responses even in his or her reflex behavior. During the course of development, certain motor patterns may dominate but different or opposing motor patterns are not totally excluded. For example, by six months of age, the baby seems to practice predominantly patterns of extension, especially when prone. When supine, however, the same baby plays frequently with patterns of flexion, i.e., raising pelvis and legs, reaching towards knees and feet.

ABNORMAL
Stereotyped movements and predominant motor patterns displayed more or less exclusively in various positions indicate central nervous system (CNS) dysfunction.

Grading of Movements

NORMAL
Grading of movements for amplitude, speed, and velocity requires integration between diverse sensory feedback systems with control centers for motor output. Motor responses must be adapted according to labyrinthine, visual,

proprioceptive, tactile, and auditory feedback. Grading of movements in space is prepared through grading of movements during weight bearing and weight shifting.

ABNORMAL

In the abnormally developing child, this learning process may be interrupted by the sensory feedback and motor control systems. Visual and auditory feedback, for example, are inaccurate and poorly integrated when the infant has poor head control. Abnormal postural alignment of the head also influences, of course, the labyrinthine feedback. Poor postural stability, such as lack of trunk control and poor proximal stabilization of the shoulder girdle, interferes with graded reaching among other motor functions. Movements are jerky and the infant overshoots when reaching. Some infants give themselves outside stability for grasping or releasing objects by leaning on arm and hand. Abnormal postural tonus also prevents the execution of graded and smooth movements. Fluctuations of tonus, involuntary movements, and tremor which may be evident at a later stage of development, make it very difficult to develop well-coordinated and efficient movement patterns. Paucity of movements or excessive, disorganized movements are further symptoms of possible CNS impairment. Sensory deficits also delay or alter motor development.

Sequencing of Movements

NORMAL

Each righting reaction is facilitatory to and may elicit other righting as well as equilibrium reactions resulting in a chain reaction or sequencing of movement patterns. Lateral head righting, for example, results in lateral righting of the trunk which, in turn, causes the limbs to assume a posture of the amphibian reaction or a balance response. The sequential activation of righting and equilibrium reactions engulfs the whole body and provides the infant with such important motor functions as change of position in space or progression.

ABNORMAL

Sequencing of movements is hampered when the development of righting and equilibrium reactions is delayed or disturbed. A smooth sequential flow of movements is often blocked by the predominance of one motor pattern or by the excessive use of one part of the body, for example, by the infant who uses arms and upper trunk as compensation for lack of motor control in legs and pelvis. A wide base of support, such as the "frog position" of the limbs or the "W sitting" position, poses a mechanical obstacle to changes of posture and disturbs the sequencing of movements. These infants then present a quite static picture which contrasts sharply with the dynamic motor behavior of a normal baby.

Integration of Primitive Reflexes

The primitive reflexes of diagnostic significance are the Moro reflex and the tonic reflexes, for example, the tonic labyrinthine reflex (TLR), the asymmetrical tonic neck reflex (ATNR), and the symmetrical tonic neck reflex (STNR).

NORMAL

These reflexes are present at birth or appear during the first weeks of life. Infants with normally developed CNS can easily move out of these primitive reflex patterns because more purposeful actions can override them. With the maturation of the CNS these primitive reflexes are modified and integrated into more complex postural reactions and are then no longer displayed in pure form.

ABNORMAL

The picture presented by some patients with CNS deficit stands in strong contrast with this description. In these patients, tonic reflexes interfere with voluntary actions. The dominance of tonic reflexes increases in time while more mature postural reflexes, such as righting and equilibrium reactions, fail to develop. Tonic reflexes are stereotyped and exaggerated when compared with the norm. Through the presence of abnormal strength and distribution of postural tonus, these primitive reflexes become increasingly abnormal. A pro-gravity pull is asserted which interferes with the development of righting against gravity.

Postural Symmetry

NORMAL

The development of symmetry and midline orientation is extremely important and a prerequisite for many perceptual skills. Integration between the two sides must take place before a higher form of laterality and reciprocality and, finally, dominance of one side can develop (three years).

ABNORMAL

Persistent postural and functional asymmetry interrupts this cycle of normal perceptual development. The lack of midline orientation and bilateral hand activities may lead to distortion of body image and body awareness and may severely hamper the ability to learn about properties of different objects.

Postural Alignment

With the influence of righting reactions, infants learn to right themselves against gravity, assuming a normal position of the head in space and maintaining or restoring proper postural alignment between head, trunk, and limbs. In each body plane there are different motor patterns associated with righting reactions.

Plane 1. Righting in the Sagittal Plane (Extension and Flexion Against Gravity)

NORMAL

Although the development of postural control starts with patterns of extension against gravity, more mature patterns of righting in the sagittal plane require coordination between axial extension and flexion. Through the progressive development of postural control of flexion against gravity, the infant is able to assume a symmetrical posture and engages in hand to hand, feet, knees, or mouth activities while supine. A combination of patterns of flexion and extension leads to mature and balanced postural alignment of head and trunk and provides proximal stability. Differentiated movements of the limbs become possible; for example, forward reach with extended elbows, or lifting of extended legs while supine.

ABNORMAL

Postural tonus. Instead of righting against gravity, the infant may sink into gravity (hypotonicity) or be pulled into gravity (hypertonicity). Progravity pull is especially strong when tonic reflexes dominate motor behavior. Hypertonicity increases the more the infant tries to move against gravity. Effort and stress have the same effect.

Coordination between flexion and extension. The fine interplay between extension and flexion is often disturbed in the presence of CNS impairment. While these infants may be able to move against gravity to some extent, postural alignment is abnormal and motor components are poorly integrated (see Chap. 4).

Dominant extensor patterns. When patterns of extension predominate, the cervical and lumbar spine are pulled into excessive lordosis. As a consequence, the head retracts while the chin juts forward. The neck cannot elongate without the development of flexion against gravity. Without the counterbalance of flexion the pelvis is pulled into an anterior tilt which interferes with the development of full hip extension. Further development of righting and balancing in all body planes is severely hampered.

Compensatory flexion. Predominant flexion frequently occurs as a compensatory pattern, especially in more upright positions such as sitting or during crawling, etc. The abnormal pull into flexion is then superimposed on early (extensor) patterns developed in prone and supine.

Plane 2.   Righting in the Frontal Plane (Lateral Flexion)

NORMAL

Proper postural alignment in the frontal plane requires lateral righting: a pattern of side flexion of neck and trunk towards the non-weightbearing side together with active elongation and extension on the weightbearing side. With progressive lateral displacement, a component of axial rotation emerges. Lateral righting is only possible when total patterns of extension and flexion are inhibited and, therefore, seems to be a significant skill in the course of development.

ABNORMAL

Lateral righting is not developed when total and synergic patterns of extension and flexion prevail. Although lateral trunk flexion is often substituted for trunk rotation, a close observation of the postural alignment reveals considerable differences in the quality and efficiency of the response when compared with a true righting response. In abnormal development, lateral flexion does not provide good postural alignment since it is often combined with predominant extension of the spine. Shoulder girdle and pelvic girdle are not aligned in the frontal plane. There is no active elongation on the weight-bearing side. However, mechanical stability is achieved in the end range of vertebral joints.

Plane 3.   Righting in the Transverse Plane (Rotation Within the Body Axis)

NORMAL

Rotation within the body axis develops with the influence of body righting on the body. It is an essential component of a wide variety of functional skills such as change of position (for example, sidelying to sitting, sitting to crawling). In addition, righting within the body axis can be observed in segmental rolling. Between prone and supine, rolling is initiated from the pelvis; between supine and prone, rolling is initiated from head and shoulders. In more upright positions, such as sitting, the development of rotation allows trunk control and frees the arms for manipulation of toys and refinement of hand function. Rotation can be combined with flexion as in equilibrium reactions or with extension as in the transition between sitting and quadruped.

ABNORMAL

Patients with CNS deficit frequently fail to develop rotation within the body axis and the resulting refined form of balancing. Side flexion of the head and trunk is often substituted and balancing requires undue effort. The infant has to rely on a broad base of support, i.e., wide abduction of the limbs, which encourages static positions. Furthermore, the arms must be used for protection against falling because of poor trunk control. Play activities and manipulation of objects are consequently restricted.

Postural Stability and Motility

Every movement displaces the center of gravity and requires postural adjustments which increase in complexity with a decrease of outside support. Controlled movement requires a counterbalance of postural stability. This postural stability must be adjusted at every phase of the movements. Efficient postural stability is, therefore, dynamic. Controlled movements of the extremities are based on proximal stability. Controlled movements of the body in space are made possible through the development of equilibrium reactions.

Dynamic Proximal Stability

NORMAL

In accordance with the cephalo to caudal and proximal to distal sequence of development, postural stability is first seen around the neck and shoulder girdle, then in the trunk, and later in the pelvic girdle. Postural stability is developed through the weight bearing. The infant can perform fine controlled movements of the upper extremities in space only after achieving stability of the shoulder girdle and trunk through activities of weight bearing and weight shifting of the upper extremities (by about five to six months of age). Controlled and isolated finger movements require, in addition, good stability of elbow and wrist. Efficient head and trunk control is made possible through the development of weight shifting through lower trunk and pelvis. Balancing activities of the lower extremities and feet require postural control of trunk and pelvis.

ABNORMAL

Lack of proximal stability causes difficulties in midline control for all body planes, i.e., proper alignment between head, shoulder, and pelvic girdle cannot be achieved. Weight shifting is often occasioned by movements of the head (head tilting towards weight bearing side or into gravity), which directly opposes proper righting, and balance reactions (head and trunk tilting against gravity). Further development of head and trunk control is consequently hampered and manipulative skills are not fully developed. Motor patterns of the lower extremities become increasingly abnormal.

Patterns of fixation. The infant who lacks proper patterns of weight shifting, righting, and balancing tries to obtain some postural stability with abnormal patterns of fixation. In contrast with normal postural stability, these patterns of fixation are static and interfere with efficient weight shifting; and in time, lead to contractures. They occur most often around shoulder and pelvic girdle and are expressed, for example, in elevation of shoulders or anterior pelvic tilt. A broad base of support, i.e., wide abduction of the limbs, may also be used for postural stability resulting again in a static posture. Another form of abnormal postural fixation occurs at distal points of the limbs, especially in the hypotonic infant who tends to stabilize by leaning on the lateral and ulnar side of hands and feet. A distal point of fixation is also achieved by crossing the feet which is often seen when the infant sits.

Equilibrium Reactions

NORMAL

While righting reactions provide postural alignment, equilibrium reactions maintain and restore balance through tonal adjustments or compensatory movements. Equilibrium reactions build on and modify righting reactions. They appear at the age of about six months and emerge first in prone, then in supine, then in sitting, in quadruped, and, finally, in standing and walking. By the time full repertoire of equilibrium reactions is achieved, the child is five to six years old. It is interesting to note that the infant is already sitting unsupported when first equilibrium reactions in prone develop. The same temporal overlapping of motor functions occurs between sitting and standing and standing and walking. Balance reactions in standing and walking emerge during the second year of life and include, in addition to proximal postural adjustments, compensatory steps in all directions as well as intrinsic, compensatory movements of forefoot and toes. During the subsequent years, postural adjustments become more refined. Equilibrium reactions consist of lateral flexion or axial rotation of head and trunk and a "reaching pattern" of the extremities. The pattern of the extremities depends on the direction of the weight shift; usually it incorporates some degree of external rotation and extension.

The subtle and quick postural adjustments of the equilibrium reactions can only occur when a high degree of differentiation of movement patterns is achieved.

ABNORMAL

Primitive and total movement patterns, limitations as to mobility, and abnormal postural tonus interfere with the performance of equilibrium reactions.

Protective Extension of the Arms

NORMAL

Protective extension of the arms is applied when other balance reactions are insufficient. Its development preceeds and partially overlaps with that of other equilibrium reactions. By about five to six months, the infant leans on slightly fisted hands when sitting unsupported. During the following weeks, greater wrist mobility develops allowing better extension of wrist and fingers with stronger extension throughout the arm. Protective extension of the arms forwards, sideways, and backwards develop between six and twelve months of age.

ABNORMAL

The infant who lacks shoulder girdle and trunk stability cannot develop efficient patterns of upper extremity weight bearing. Also, protective extension of the arms is normally combined with appropriate head righting. Any delay or disturbance in the development of righting reactions interferes with the development of appropriate protective extension of the arms.

Dissociation of Movements (Mature Versus Primitive Motor Patterns)

NORMAL

The ability to combine components of different patterns, such as patterns of flexion and extension, requires an inhibitory control and develops, therefore, only gradually with progressive CNS maturation. Total motor patterns must be inhibited for isolated and differentiated movements to occur. Dissociation of total motor patterns allows formation of a vast variety of new movement patterns and provides the postural mechanism for all skillful motor activities.

A very primitive and preparatory function of dissociation may be seen in the ATNR-posture where each side of the body assumes a different pattern. Righting reactions and the amphibian reaction evolve with further development of inhibitory control and suppress this. Some other patterns of dissociation have been described in Chapter 4.

Differentiation of proximal movements preceeds those occuring distally. Progression is cephalo to caudal; therefore, dissociation between movements of head, shoulder girdle, and trunk—as seen for example, during lateral weight shifting in prone on elbows or hands—occurs before the infant is able to dissociate pelvic movements from movements of the trunk Such dissociation enables the infant, for example, to rotate the pelvis back during rolling or when prone so as to sit. Dissociation between movements of leg and pelvis express an even later stage of development and changes, for example, the gait patterns eliminating the pronounced lateral hiking of the pelvis while the hip flexes during the swing phase. The pattern of heel strike as seen in the mature gait pattern indicates differentiation of movement patterns throughout the whole body. As with the development of rotation, these skills must be conquered in each position. For instance, dissociation of movements of hip, knee, and ankle is applied in prone, then while sitting and crawling before it can be incorporated into the mature gait pattern.

ABNORMAL

The development of dissociation and differentiation of movement patterns is disturbed in combination with sensorimotor deficits. Primitive and synergic motor patterns persist and become increasingly inefficient for higher and complex motor tasks. Compensatory and abnormal motor patterns emerge,

especially when the infant assumes more upright positions, and the gap between normal and abnormal motor behavior becomes increasingly larger.

PRIMARY ABNORMAL PATTERNS AND
COMPENSATORY ABNORMAL PATTERNS

Differentiation between primary abnormal patterns and abnormal patterns
that compensate for them is important in designing the treatment program.
An approach concerned only with patterns of compensation may reinforce
and increase the original abnormality which in turn increases the necessity
for patterns of compensation; for example, emphasizing extension in the infant who uses compensatory flexion in order to overcome abnormal extension may only elicit more compensatory flexion.

Abnormal development follows basically the course of normal development in its cephalo to caudal progression. Primary and initial signs of abnormality, therefore, often include a disturbance of head righting and an interference in shoulder girdle stability, depending on the type of CNS damage.
Also, as in normal development, patterns of extension emerge first and seem
to dominate the motor behavior for a prolonged time. Quality and distribution of extension, however, differ from that seen in normal development (see
Chap. 4).

Compensatory patterns emerge mostly in more upright positions and with
attempts at locomotion. The earliest and most frequently seen consists of
abnormal flexion of upper trunk and neck combined with shoulder elevation
and scapular protraction. Flexor hypertonicity may then be superimposed on
abnormal extensor tonus.

CONTRACTURES AND DEFORMITIES

The infant who is restricted to few patterns of posture and movement is
likely to display limited mobility and may develop contractures and even deformities. A test for mobility is applied based on the suspected effects of
predominant patterns of posture and movements. To distinguish between
movement restrictions due to hypertonicity and the presence of true contractures the infant must be tested while well-aligned.

Some of the most obvious factors for the development of contractures and
deformities are dominating tonic reflexes (Figs. 1a,1b).

Extensor hypertonicity eventually causes shortening of hip extensors
(Figs. 2a,2b). Retraction of the shoulders leads to a fixation between the
scapula and humerus and, eventually, a winging of the scapula whenever the
arm is raised (Fig. 3).

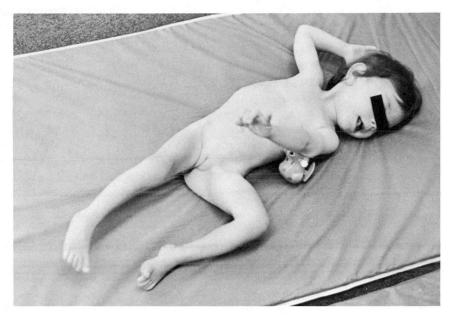

Figure 1a A hypertonic pattern of adduction and internal rotation of the right hip, plantarflexion, and inversion of the right foot is elicited and constantly reinforced by the dominating influence of the ATNR toward the left and may lead to subluxation or dislocation of the right hip.

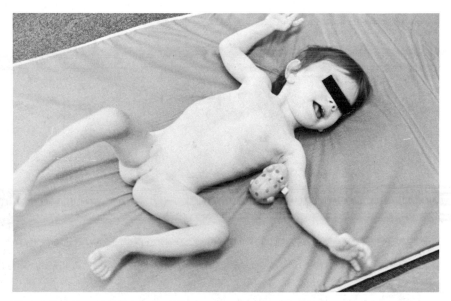

Figure 1b Restricted hip mobility is also demonstrated when the hips are flexed.

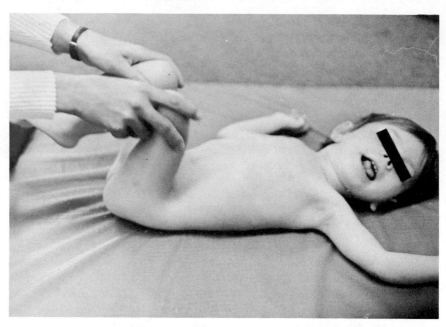

Figure 2a Restricted mobility in hip flexion results from predominant extensor hypertonicity.

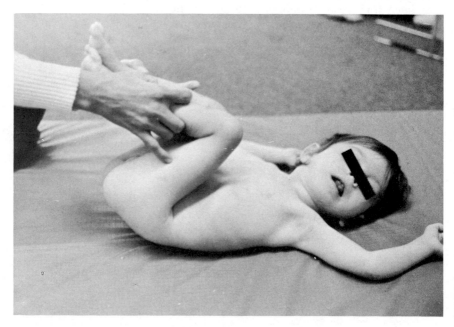

Figure 2b When the legs are elevated beyond ninety degrees, the pelvis is pulled off the support, indicating shortened hip extensors.

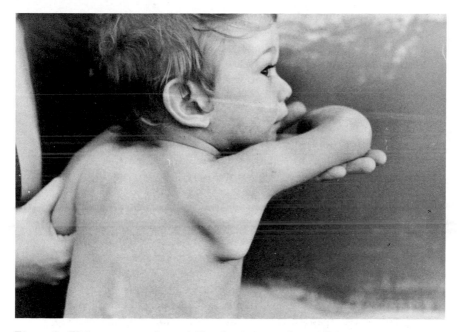

Figure 3 With poor scapular stability, humerus and scapula move as a unit. In time, muscles between scapula and humerus become progressively shorter, leading to excessive winging of the scapula whenever the arm is raised (compare with Fig. 34c, Chap. 4).

Predominant extensor tonus and a habitual pattern of neck retraction interfere with flexion and elongation of the cervical spine, even in a very young infant. Restricted mobility occurs also in other areas of the spine and effects movements of trunk and pelvis.

Although the hypotonic child tends to display hypermobility in most joints, some contractures may develop due to habitual posturing. For example, a persistent pattern of flexion and abduction of the legs, so typical for the hypotonic patient, may interfere with full hip extension and adduction and may pose severe problems when the child attempts to stand or walk.

The STNR-posture, which is used by many patients extensively for sitting ("W sitting") and for crawling, soon results in flexor contractures of the legs and may seriously interfere with the development of independent standing and walking.

These are only a few examples. A variety of compensatory patterns emerge, especially in more upright positions and with attempts at locomotion; their impact must be evaluated on an individual basis.

Abnormal patterns of posture and movements as well as abnormal postural tonus can cause severe deformities. Dislocations and subluxations, as mentioned above, are certainly not restricted to the hip joint. In addition to scoliosis, other deformities of the ribcage occur, especially in the infant who does not assume antigravity positions and therefore develops a rather flat and broad rib cage. These deformities can have a severe impact on patterns of respiration and phonation.

In order to recommend appropriate methods of prevention, the therapy evaluation must aim to uncover abnormal motor behavior that may be enforcing the development of contractures and deformities.

BIBLIOGRAPHY

André-Thomas, and Autgaerden, S.: Locomotion From Pre- To Post-Natal Life. Clinics in Developmental Medicine, No. 24. London, The Spastics Society Medical Education and Information Unit in association with Heinemann, 1966.

André-Thomas, Chesni, I., and Saint-Anne Dargassies, S.: The Neurological Examination Of The Infant. Clinics in Developmental Medicine, No. 1, London, The Spastic Society Medical Education and Information Unit in association with Heinemann, 1960.

Bèbe, M.: Mi Hijo Su Primer Año. Buenos Aires, Sigmar, 1979.

Blankenstein, M. V., Welbergen, U. R., and Haas, J. H. de: Le Développment Du Nourisson. Paris, Presses Universitaires de France, 1962.

Bly, L.: The Components Of Normal And Abnormal Movement During The First Year Of Life. Proceedings from Development of Movement in Infants, May 1980. Division of Physical Therapy, University of North Carolina, Chapel Hill, N.C., 1981.

Bobath, B.: Abnormal Postural Reflex Activity Caused By Brain Lesions. (2nd ed.). London, Heinemann, 1971.

Bobath, B., and Bobath, K.: Motor Development In The Different Types Of Cerebral Palsy. London, Heinemann, 1975.

Bobath, K.: The Motor Deficit In Patients With Cerebral Palsy. Clinics in Developmental Medicine, No. 23. London, Heinemann, 1966.

Bosma, J.: Form and Function in the infant's mouth and pharynx. In Third Symposium on Oral Sensation and Perception. Bosma, J. (Ed.). Springfield, Thomas, 3-29, 1972.

Bower, T. G. R.: Development In Infancy. San Francisco, Freeman, 1974.

Brazelton, T. B.: Infants And Mothers, Differences In Development. New York, Dell, 1969.

Brazelton, T. B.: Neonatal Behavioral Assessment Scale. Clinics in Developmental Medicine, No. 50. London, The Spastics Society Medical Education and Information Unit in association with Heinemann, 1973.

Brazelton, T. B.: Toddlers And Parents, A Declaration Of Independence. New York, Delacorte Press, 1974.

Caplan, F. (gen. ed.): The First Twelve Months Of Life, Your Baby's Growth Month by Month, New York, Grosset & Dunlap, 1973.

Caplan, F., and Caplan, T.: The Second Twelve Months Of Life, A Kaleidoscope Of Growth. New York, Grosset & Dunlap, 1979.

Capute, A., Accardo, P., Vining, E., Rubenstein, J., and Harryman, S.: Primitive Reflex Profile. Monographs In Developmental Pediatrics, Vol. 1. Baltimore, University Park Press, 1978.

Casaer, P.: Postural Behavior In Newborn Infants. Philadelphia, Lippincott, 1979.

Gesell, A., Amatruda, C. S.: Developmental Diagnosis. Normal And Abnormal Child Development. New York, Hoeber, 1947.

Haberfellner, H.: Zur Frueherkennung Der Cerebralen Bewegungsstoerungen. *Oester. Aerzt.* 32:1092–1095, 1977.

Hochleitner, M.: Pathologische Motorische Entwicklung Bei Cerebralparese, Motoskopische Diagnostik. Goettingen, Institut fuer den Wissenschaftlichen Film, C 1107, 1973.

Illingworth, R. S.: The Development Of The Infant And Young Child, Normal And Abnormal (3rd ed.). London, Livingstone, 1967.

Ingram, T. T. S.: The new approach to early diagnosis of handicaps in childhood. *Dev. Med. Child Neurol.* 11:279–290, 1969.

Koeng, E.: Fruehdiagnose Cerebraler Laehmungen. *Paediatr. Fortbldg. Praxis* 1:37–44, 1962.

Koeng, E.: Frueherfassung Cerebraler Bewegungsstoerungen. *Paediatr. Fortbldg. Praxs* 33:1–14, 1972.

Milani-Comparetti, A., Gidoni, E. A.: Pattern analysis of motor development and its disorders. *Dev. Med. Child Neurol.* 9:625–630, 1967.

Milani-Comparetti, A., Gidoni, E. A.: Routine development examination in normal and retarded children. *Dev. Med. Child Neurol.* 9:631–638, 1967.

Paine, R. S.: Early recognition of neuromotor disabilities in infants with low birth weight. *Dev. Med. Child Neurol.* 11:455–459, 1969

Peiper, A.: Cerebral Function In Infancy And Childhood. New York, Consultants Bureau, 1963.

Prechtl, H., Beintema, D.: The Neurological Examination Of The Full-Term Newborn Infant. Clinics in Developmental Medicine, No. 12. London, The Spastics Society Medical Education and Information Unit in association with Heinemann, 1964.

Rosenblith, J. F.: Behavioral Examination Of The Neonate. Proceedings from

Comprehensive Management of Infants at Risk for CNS Deficit, May, 1974. Division of Physical Therapy, University of North Carolina, Chapel Hill, 1975.

Saint-Anne Dargassies, S.: Neurodevelopmental symptoms during the first year of life. *Dev. Med. Child Neurol.* 14:235–246, 1972.

Saint-Anne Dargassies, S.: Neurological Development In The Full-Term And Premature Neonate. Amsterdam, Elsevier, 1977.

Stern, F.: The reflex development of the infant. *Am. J. Occup. Ther.* 25:155–158, 1971.

Touwen, B.: Neurological Development In Infancy. Clinics in Developmental Medicine, No. 58. London, Heinemann, 1976.

Weisz, St.: Studies in equilibrium reaction. *J. Nerv. Ment. Dis.* 88:150–162, 1938.

White, B.: The First Three Years Of Life. Englewood Cliffs, N.J., Prentice-Hall, 1975.

Wilson, J.: Developmental reflex test. In Vulpe, S.: The Vulpe Assessment Battery. National Institute on Mental Retardation, Toronto, 1977.

6

Neurodevelopmental Assessment of Infants: Procedures

OVERVIEW

Examination and screening procedures preceding the therapy evaluation avail the therapist with some background information of the patient (see also Chapters 2 and 3). When the diagnosis is not sufficiently clear, identification of suspect central nervous system (CNS) dysfunction and consequent referral for further assessment are based on some of the following symptoms.

1. Stereotyped behavior, paucity of movement, excessive and disorganized movement
2. Poor control and alignment of head, face not in vertical plane, hyperextension of head and neck
3. Consistent elevation of shoulder girdle, scapular protraction or retraction
4. Pronounced anterior or posterior pelvic tilt, incomplete hip extension
5. Hypotonicity with "frog posture" of limbs
6. Hypertonicity—pulled into gravity

7. Low proximal tonus combined with high distal tonus, consistent fisting of hands with pronation, and internal rotation of arms

8. Pronounced extensor patterns of legs with adduction of hips and clawing of toes

9. Feeding problems

The therapy assessment aims at analyzing in depth the quality of sensorimotor functions, adaptive and feeding behavior. A detailed analysis of normal and abnormal development is presented in Chapter 4. In this chapter, an interdisciplinary model for the therapy assessment is presented; developmental skills and the quality of underlying motor patterns are evaluated in various positions; and an assessment of adaptive behavior and a detailed feeding evaluation are described. Recommendations for an evaluation report and a motor evaluation form are also included.

For the assessment to be a meaningful tool for treatment and management programming, it must go beyond a mere description of presented behavior. Instead, the therapist attempts to determine how different responses affect each other. It is important to find the primary component in a chain reaction of abnormal responses and to determine the most important postural mechanisms and motor components that would allow more appropriate function. The therapist should at all times be guided by the infant's behavior. Only then will the assessment be a truly investigative process and a helpful tool for designing a meaningful treatment program. Concepts and basic principles underlying this assessment approach are listed in Chapter 5.

INITIAL EVALUATION

Organization

Experts in different disciplines assess different sections of the infant's behavior. For a better understanding of the total situation of patient and family, close communication between the different disciplines is mandatory. Implementation of the team concept in the initial therapy assessment or screening seems preferable to separate evaluations by each specialist. Different models of the team approach are practiced and must be adjusted to the special circumstances. The therapy team includes physical, occupational, and speech therapists who collaborate closely with the physician, social worker, home service staff, psychologist, and teacher. At least one team member should evaluate the patient and family members in their home.

When the initial evaluation is carried out by a whole team, it will not be complete and detailed. The team aims to gather the most important information in each area of development: sensorimotor behavior, feeding, prespeech, and language development, sensory functions, social, emotional, and cognitive development. The initial evaluation serves to determine major problems and areas requiring immediate intervention. Recommendations for further evaluation in specific areas will result from this.

The combined information of all team members outlines the infant's abilities and areas for concern, allowing the recommendations for intervention programs to be tailored to the individual needs of patient and family. This information must be presented to the family as soon as possible. The multidisciplinary team evaluation makes it possible to reduce to a minimum the time the family must wait for evaluation results, which can produce severe anxiety if it is long.

Interviewing the Parent

At the beginning of the session, the team should obtain information from the accompanying parent about the infant's behavior at home, possible difficulties in care taking, the family's major concerns related to the infant's deficits, and, finally, the family's expectations for their child's future.

Method of Assessment

The sensorimotor evaluation is carried out by observing spontaneous behavior, eliciting specific responses, and assessing the patient's potential for more mature postural reactions as facilitated through specific handling.

While interviewing the parent, the therapist establishes some rapport with both the parent and the infant. Interaction between the infant and the parent is observed as well as other adaptive behavior (see Chapter 5). Postural reactions to being carried and undressed are assessed. The parent is then asked to place the child on the mat for further observation of spontaneous behavior. Reactions to the separation from the parent, interest in and interaction with toys, as well as motor behavior are observed. Sensorimotor behavior is described as evidenced by motor functions and the quality of motor patterns as described in Chapter 5. Special emphasis is placed on righting reactions and equilibrium responses.

When placed on a mat, the infant is allowed to move without help and in this way to show whole movement repertoire without extensive prompting. Alternatively, the therapist sets up the environment by selectively placing toys around, thus challenging to the very limit, the child's available motor abilities and skills.

EVALUATION OF MOTOR DEVELOPMENT

Motor Behavior in Different Positions

Spontaneous motor functions and specific postural reactions are observed and elicited in a variety of positions. Special attention is focused on abnormal motor patterns which are repeated in various positions. Criteria for normal and abnormal sensorimotor behavior and some respective examples have been discussed in detail in Chapter 4 and 5.

Supine

The extent and quality of spontaneous posture and movements are recorded before the therapist handles the infant.

   The infant's predominant postural asymmetry should be carefully evaluated. Asymmetrical posturing of the limbs is related to proximal patterns, i.e., turning of the head, posture of shoulder girdle, pelvis and trunk. Asymmetry of movements, such as reaching, grasping, kicking, etc., is easy to detect.

   Predominant extensor tonus is expressed in hyperlordosis of the cervical and lumbar spine, but also in scapular adduction and retraction of the arms. Elevation of the shoulders often accompanies poor head control. It should be noted if the head position determines body posture and oral posture or if the infant is able to differentiate movements of head, shoulder girdle, and trunk. Primitive or abnormal posture of the limbs, such as "frog position," is recorded.

   Prevalence of static postures or the presence of movements such as handplay, hands to feet, and their respective quality are described. Ability or disability to move out of the supine position is reported and the patterns used are noted, i.e., segmental rolling, primitive, total, or abnormal patterns. Some infants may use "bridging" and abnormal extension for progression while supine.

   The therapist then handles the infant for a more precise assessment of postural tonus. The head position and its influence on the distribution of tonus are closely observed. Restrictions of mobility and contractures can be investigated at the same time. The infant's reactions to handling by the therapist are also interpreted as to tactile sensitivity.

   Full overhead extension of the arms may be difficult to achieve and may cause excessive winging of the scapula and compensatory hyperlordosis of the lumbar spine. Mobility of the hips is tested. A symmetrical position of the pelvis must be ensured during these tests to determine accurately the range of mobility. Repetitive and brisk abduction of the hips may reveal underlying hypertonicity even when the basic tonus is low. Dorsiflexion of the ankle may be reduced due to abnormal extensor tonus. The degree of elongation of the neck can be evaluated by elevating pelvis and legs while flexing the spine. Head righting and active flexion against gravity are evaluated by pulling the infant by his or her hands to a sitting position.

The infant who does not spontaneously bring the hands together or to his or her mouth, feet, etc., is encouraged to reach with both hands for a toy held in midline. Assistance is given when required. A noise-making toy or crumpling a piece of paper is used to test hearing and auditory attention. A toy is also used to determine the ability for focusing and visual tracking. Toys of different textures are used to investigate tactile sensitivity.

Tracking may cause the infant to roll from supine to prone. Otherwise, the therapist facilitiates rolling from the infant's legs while assessing whether proper head and trunk righting as well as rotation are applied.

Prone

The assessment in prone starts again with an observation of spontaneous posture and movements, such as reaching, rolling, creeping, etc. The degree and quality of extension against gravity is related to chronological age (see Chap. 4). If, during rolling towards prone, the infant's arms get stuck under his or her body, the therapist facilitates weight shifting from pelvis or trunk to allow the infant to free his or her arms. When the pull into flexion is strong, the therapist places the infant's arms forward for propping. This is a good opportunity to assess tonus and mobility of shoulder girdle and arms. Lateral righting, the ability to shift weight, and to reach for objects is evaluated in the puppy position and/or while propped on the hands. Assistance may be necessary to stabilize the pelvis in children lacking hip extension.

Using a toy, the therapist tries to elicit progression which can take the form of pivoting, while leaning on the hands, pushing backwards (caudally) on extended arms, rolling, or creeping on the belly. Any distinct asymmetry (use of limbs, head position, torsion of trunk and pelvis) is recorded. The excessive use of arms, as in "commando crawling" (belly creeping) may result in tight extension and adduction of the legs. Where spontaneous belly crawling is not achievable, the therapist facilitates a shift of weight from trunk or pelvis to elicit the amphibian reaction. This is a preparatory function for crawling; where abnormal tonus prevails, the infant will fail to achieve a sufficient degree of dissociation of movements.

Quadruped

When appropriate, chronologically and developmentally, the infant is encouraged to assume the quadruped position and to crawl on hands and knees. When balance and dissociation of movements are poor, both hips are kept in pronounced flexion during crawling, and more or less tight dorsiflexion of the ankle may be present. When the hypertonicity is strong, crawling takes the form of bunny hopping. Rotation and counterrotation between shoulder girdle and pelvis cannot occur as long as the spine is excessively flexed or extended and as long as the legs are in pronounced abduction. Upper extremity weight bearing is assessed for pronounced scapular protraction and elevation, internal rotation of shoulders, insufficient or excessive extension of the arms, and fisting of the hands. Any postural asymmetry is recorded.

Progression

Other forms of progression, such as rolling, belly crawling, etc., are evaluated for movement flow, postural alignment, and postural–functional symmetry.

Sitting

The sitting position and the ability to assume sitting are evaluated. Has the infant sufficient proximal stability to use the hands freely for manipulation? When necessary, minimal assistance is given by the examiner. The sitting posture is analyzed for postural alignment between pelvis, shoulder girdle, and head as viewed from the front (lateral flexion of the spine, lateral tilt of shoulder girdle and pelvis), from the side (flexion or extension of upper and/or lower trunk and hips, anterior or posterior pelvic tilt), and in the transverse plane (torsion of pelvis, shoulder girdle, and trunk, and turning of head). Does the infant sit on the ischial tuberosities or the sacrum? The posture of the lower extremities is evaluated for predominantly primitive (flexion, abduction, external rotation of hips, flexion of knees), abnormal (flexion, adduction, internal rotation of hips), or mature and differentiated patterns.

Are the feet used for patterns of fixation? Are the arms held in high guard posture? It should be recorded whether the arms are used for propping or whether they are free for manipulation; there may also be abnormal posturing of the upper extremities such as scapular protraction and elevation, internal rotation of the shoulders, etc.

Symmetry of weight bearing on the hips is best evaluated by placing both hands under the patient's pelvis. Righting and equilibrium reactions as well as protective extension of the arms can be elicited while the therapist shifts the center of gravity to either side and backwards or forwards, either from the pelvis or from the trunk. The child with sufficient sitting balance is placed on a movable surface (tiltboard, ball). Sitting balance and rotation within the body axis can also be elicited when the therapist encourages the infant to reach for toys in all directions, including backwards. This may lead to a change of position from sitting to quadruped, side sitting, or prone. Degree of control and quality of movements are noted.

The infant who lacks trunk control and dissociation of movements often learns to sit unsupported by sitting between the heels and thus achieves a broad and stable base (W sitting). In these infants, sitting balance and posture are to be evaluated in longleg sitting as outlined above.

Upper Extremity Function

Activities of reaching, grasping, and releasing are evaluated as to accuracy, voluntary control, and refinement. Some children may achieve stability for release and manipulation of objects by leaning on the hand. Weight bearing and weight shifting are assessed in prone, quadruped, and sitting. In all positions, the therapist may manipulate the infant from pelvis and trunk to achieve the desired weight distribution. Protective extension can be tested in sitting.

Standing and Walking

Abnormal patterns observed in lower positions may become even more pronounced when the child stands or walks. The emphasis of evaluation is on postural alignment, base of support, postural control, and the patterns of weight bearing and weight shifting. Some typical patterns of standing and walking have been described in Chapter 4.

Supported standing is assessed in the nonambulatory infant following the same criteria.

Elicited Primitive and Postural Reflexes

A test for positive and negative supporting as well as the parachute reaction of the legs can be combined with the test for lateral righting of head and trunk in vertical suspension. The Landau reaction is tested in ventral suspension.

The influence of the Moro reflex, where present, is usually noticeable during the evaluation and may, therefore, not require a specific test. Similarly, tonic reflex posturing and its interference with appropriate postural reactions is expressed in spontaneous behavior. A specific test for these reflexes may therefore be superfluous.

MOTOR EVALUATION REPORT

The therapist should record motor patterns in as much detail as possible to identify consistent and dominant abnormal reactions. For a clear and meaningful report, however, this information must be condensed, categorized, and interpreted. Chapter 5 contains suggestions on how to categorize behavior. The therapist's interpretation of major and primary deficiencies determines

emphasis of treatment and management plan. Recommendations for intended
programming should also be included.

When the report is kept in a descriptive format, a consistent outline should
be followed at each subsequent reevaluation to allow a comparison. A checklist evaluation form may narrow the observation to the items listed while
overlooking some of the infant's most important behaviors. Checklists also
make it difficult to investigate how different behaviors correlate with each
other on an individual basis. The Motor Evaluation Form presented here (see
Appendix) is intended as a guide, leaving room for adaptations to the individual needs of each patient.

EVALUATION OF ORAL DEVELOPMENT
AND FEEDING SKILLS

This part of the evaluation consists of: a brief postural assessment as it relates
to oral function, an analysis of feeding patterns, and an oral examination.

Postural Assessment

Postural reactions which influence feeding skills include the degree and quality of head control, trunk control, and shoulder girdle stability; the quality
and distribution of postural tonus; and the dominance of tonic reflexes.

These postural reactions can be, to a great extent, assessed while the infant
is still on the parent's lap. The alignment between head, shoulders, and pelvis
should be described and related to oral and facial posture. Retraction of head
and shoulders, or abnormal and dominating extension throughout the body,
is often accompanied by open mouth posture, abnormal tongue posture,
drooling, and, possibly, retraction of the lips. Abnormal flexor tonus may
underlie lip pursing and tightly closed jaws. Consistent postural and oral
asymmetry should be noted. The therapist observes whether the infant puts
hands or objects into his or her mouth.

This postural assessment can be combined with an interview of the parent
about feeding procedures and difficulties. The parent is asked about the usual
feeding position, types and approximate amount of food consumed, types of
utensils used, and the length of the feeding procedure.

To allow a more detailed and qualitative assessment of feeding behavior,
the parent is asked to feed the infant.

Observation of Feeding Patterns

Position

While the parent feeds the infant, the therapist notes the infant's position
and possible impact on the oral function. Is the infant reclined, and how far?

Or is the baby seated upright? Alignment of head, trunk, and pelvis, and obvious tightness in the shoulder girdle and neck area are documented. Are patterns of abnormal extension or asymmetry reinforced by the infant's position or by the parent's approach? How much support is given and is it sufficient?

Sucking

Sucking is analyzed for efficiency, loss of liquid, and coordination between sucking, swallowing, and breathing. The movement patterns of jaw, tongue, and lips are also observed.

Normally developing infants progress through three different stages of sucking behavior. The neonate approximates the lips tightly around the nipple. Due to this seal, the rhythmical raising and lowering of tongue and jaw create negative pressure in the oral cavity which assists in emptying the nipple. A decrease of flexor tonus and a relative increase of extensor tonus reduce this tight approximation around the nipple soon thereafter. The baby then relies mostly on the suckling pattern where the nipple is stroked with tongue movements of protraction and retraction. With increased postural stability and better coordination between patterns of flexion and extension, the baby is again able to create good lip sealing and a negative pressure to suck on the nipple with controlled upwards and downwards movements of the tongue.

Abnormally developing infants seem to maintain a suckling pattern for a prolonged time. This is combined with an abnormal swallowing pattern in which the tongue protrudes between the lips and pushes the liquid out.

For infants who are bottle fed, the type of nipple, ease of liquid flow, and consistency of liquid are described.

Cup Drinking

The pattern of cup drinking changes during normal development. While initial attempts at about five months of age still reflect a sucking pattern, increased lip action gradually transforms the sucking action into a sipping motion. Traces of sucking behavior are seen in children up to two years of age and are expressed in a pattern of "chewing on the cup." This is overcome when the child achieves a high degree of dissociation of jaw, tongue, and lip movements, allowing good jaw stabilization.

Abnormally developing children often apply primitive or abnormal sucking patterns to cup drinking. Frequently, the cup is placed too far into the mouth, aggravating lip retraction and/or biting on the cup.

As well as evaluating the drinking pattern, the therapist should note the size of the cup and the liquid used.

Spoon Feeding

As with cup drinking, the young infant uses sucking patterns when starting to take food from the spoon, making initial attempts at spoon feeding messy. During the later months of the first year, the baby gradually develops the ability to remove the food from the spoon with the lips. With intrinsic movements, the tongue gathers the food into a bolus, transfers it back to be swallowed, and leans against the alveolar ridge during swallowing to seal off the oral cavity preventing food from escaping.

A primitive or abnormal suck interferes with successful spoon feeding. Instead of taking the food off the spoon with the lips, the tongue thrusts forward and the lips retract. Scraping the food along the teeth or gums further reinforces retraction of the lips. During swallowing, the tongue may protrude and push food out. The hypersensitive infant may bite down on the spoon in an uncontrolled tonic motion. Hyperextension of the jaw may occur in response to the approaching spoon. When dealing with severe feeding and swallowing problems, some parents may resort to "bird feeding," i.e., the infant's head is tilted far back and the food is dropped into the throat; thus the infant gets no sensory input for actively removing the food from the spoon, nor for transferring the food back with the tongue to be swallowed (Fig. 1).

The therapist should also note the type and shape of the spoon as well as which food is presented to the infant.

Biting and Chewing

The development of biting and chewing begins before the infant has acquired molars. By about six to seven months of age, when the infant has gained good head control and some trunk stability is attained, the infant starts to take solid food for chewing. At that time, the primitive up and down movement of the bite reflex is modified. For biting, the mandible moves forward while the jaw opens, and slides backwards along and behind the upper gums or teeth to tear off a piece of food. With the emergence of tongue lateralization, the food is then transported to the chewing surface and is fenced there between tongue and cheek during the chewing action. Gradually, the chewing motion incorporates a rotary component. After the food has been sufficiently ground and moistened with saliva, the tongue moves it posteriorly to be swallowed. Primitive sucking and biting reflexes are suppressed and the gag reflex decreases and is no longer elicited from the frontal third of the oral cavity.

Persistence of infantile feeding reflexes inhibits lateralization of the tongue and the development of rotary movements of the jaw. As a consequence, the food cannot be brought to and held on the biting surface. Instead, it is maintained in the mouth until it is softened and can be sucked down. Frequently, much of the food is pushed out by the tongue or accumulates on the palate.

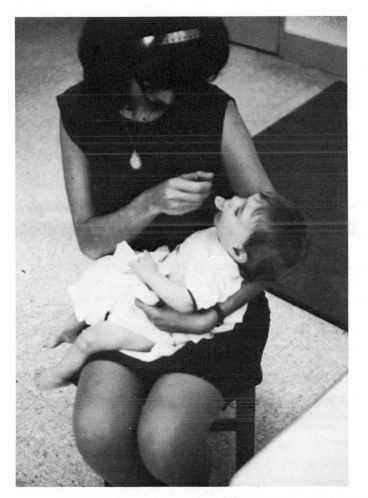

Figure 1 This is a poor but frequently used feeding posture. With the head tilted so far back into extension, it is very difficult to achieve mouth closure and proper swallowing patterns. Instead of the tongue transferring the food back, the food glides back by gravity ("bird feeding"). This feeding position does not allow the infant to develop mature and controlled feeding patterns. (From *The Infant with Cerebral Palsy: An Approach to Identification, Management, and Treatment,* A. L. Scherzer. Private printing, New York, 1973).

During the assessment of biting and chewing, the therapist focuses on the presence of mature, dissociated oral movements or on the dominance of reflex behavior and abnormal swallowing patterns. Disturbed oral function may also lead to frequent chocking on food. Vomiting during or soon after feeding is another problem which requires attention. It interferes with the infant's nourishment and may present a real danger because of possible aspiration of vomitus.

Self-Feeding

When starting to eat solids, the infant also begins to fingerfeed. At that time the lack of refined manipulative skills causes babies to push the food from the palm into the mouth rather than using a controlled placement with their fingers. By fifteen to eighteen months, the baby is able to handle a cup and a spoon with some help and supervision; and by two years of age, the child can handle food with moderate spilling.

The infant with CNS impairment may show a significant developmental delay in this area. Lack of sufficient head control and poor trunk and shoulder girdle stability require that the arms be used for support. The child who can free his or her arms but is restricted to total patterns fails to achieve graded supination of the forearm while approaching the mouth. In the last phase, the spoon or cup must be held stable while the head moves forward and the lips grab utensil and food. The handicapped child may not reach this level of motor control. In fingerfeeding, the infant may not be able to hold the food between the fingers; release may only be possible when leaning the hand against the face, thus pushing the food into the mouth in a primitive or abnormal fashion. When evaluating self-feeding, it is important to note whether the effort involved results in abnormal facial and oral tonus.

Observation of a feeding session gives also a general impression of the interaction between parent and infant, their degree of tension, and their way of coping with any difficulties.

Oral Examination

This aspect of the evaluation permits a selective and systematic investigation of those oral functions which seem to underlie the disturbed feeding behavior as displayed during the feeding session. The information obtained through the oral examination should give the therapist a more complete understanding of the patient's oral development.

A relaxed, comfortable, and symmetrical position must be chosen. Examining the infant in different positions may reveal different aspects of the abnormality of oral responses, and helps to determine the optimal function.

The oral examination includes:

Description of oral posture, tonus, and structure

Description of oral sensitivity to selective sensory stimuli

Test for oral reflexes

An assessment of vegetative breathing as it relates to swallowing and feeding

Posture, Tonus, and Structure

As in the postural evaluation, the oral examination starts with an observation of spontaneous posture and movement. Some of this information was already gathered while the infant was still on the parent's lap. However, a different picture may be presented when the baby is well-positioned and optimally supported.

Posture and tonus of cheeks, lips, and tongue should be evaluated at rest, during different stages of excitement, and during function, for example, during vocalization. The examiner should record mandibular posture and movements for protraction, retraction, depression, and lateral deviation. In addition to a possible asymmetry of the jaw, there may also be asymmetrical posturing of the tongue. It is noted whether spontaneous jaw and lip closure is present, or whether the mouth is kept open and the infant is drooling. The degree of grading of oral movements is described.

Abnormal tonus is expressed in facial and oral motions. Hypertonicity is reflected in a lack of facial and oral movements. The lips are tense and often retracted; the tongue may be retracted or elevated. The hypertonic tongue may also be elongated and thrust forward with a pointed tip. The hypotonic infant is characterized by a paucity of facial expressions, but the posture differs. Cheeks and lips are floppy, the tongue is flat and broad, and rests either on the floor of the mouth or interdentally. Fluctuations of tonus and involuntary movements create exaggerated grimacing which is typical of the athetoid patient.

For a more accurate evaluation of oral tonus, the examiner places one finger between cheeks and gums, as well as between lips and gums and touches the tongue to feel the degree of tension. It must be considered that touching the perioral and oral area provides a strong stimulus, possibly leading to a substantial increase of tonus. Also, it may not be acceptable to all patients and a resistance towards the intrusive touch by a stranger must be respected.

For the intraoral examination, a facial grasp for adequate control of the infant's mandibular movements is recommended. A detailed description of the different facial grasps can be found in Chapter 7 (Jaw Control).

The condition of the gums should be observed initially. Hyperplasia and swollen gums are often present in infants taking anticonvulsive medication. A description of the occlusion and condition of the teeth follows. Tongue thrusting and abnormal sucking patterns contribute to malocclusions, such as open bite, overbite, and cross bite. These, in turn, may aggravate abnormal biting and chewing patterns. The condition and shape of teeth are frequently impaired in combination with severe tongue thrusting and abnormal sucking patterns.

Hard and soft palates are examined for gross deviations which may influence food intake. An extremely narrow, high arched palate does not provide sufficient room to house the tongue which consequently rests interdentally. The abnormal tongue position interferes with normal patterns of swallowing, where the tongue leans against the alveolar ridge. The normal position of the tongue against the alveolar ridge seems to form a stimulating force for the maintenance of the proper arch width in the maxilla. Structure and tonus of the soft palate affect swallowing. Abnormal tonus or congenital malformations, e.g., cleft palate, may affect sucking and swallowing. When, during swallowing, the soft palate is not moved into apposition with the posterior wall of the pharynx to seal off the nasal cavity, food or liquid may escape to the nasal passages and aspiration may occur.

Sensitivity

Sensory stimuli within and around the mouth elicit a chain reaction of feeding reflexes in the normal baby. Efficient feeding behavior depends on and is regulated by accurate oral sensory feedback. The hypersensitive child reacts to stimuli of touch, taste, smell, and temperature with abnormal tension of lips, cheeks, and tongue. Retraction of the head and abnormal extension throughout the body may follow.

Deficiency of sensory feedback impairs oral function and needs close investigation. Observation of the feeding process reveals how the infant reacts to different stimuli. To appreciate more subtle tonal changes, the therapist selectively touches the oral and perioral area.

Reflexes

Perioral and oral touch also represent the stimulus for different oral reflexes. The reflexes to be tested are the rooting, suck-swallowing, bite, and gag reflexes.

The rooting reflex is present at birth and allows the infant to move the head in search for food long before head control is established. As a stimulus, the infant is stroked on the cheeks, above and below the lips. The reflex is positive when the infant pouts lips, protrudes tongue, and turns head in the direction of the stimulus. In the infant with CNS impairment, the rooting reflex may be particularly pronounced, inhibiting more selective lip action and contributing to asymmetries of lips, jaw, and tongue.

Associated with the rooting reflex is the suck–swallowing reflex which is elicited when a finger or nipple is brought into the mouth. A description of this reflex is discussed in the section "Observation of Feeding Patterns." At this point the therapist examines whether sucking is a voluntary response or a reflexive behavior.

The bite reflex is also present during the early months of life and is elicited by touching the gums to the side or on the biting surface. The infant reacts with a straight upward–downward movement of the mandible. In normal development, this reflex behavior is altered by the emergence of mature biting and chewing. In abnormal development, the bite reflex is easily elicited and may persist, interfering with the development of mature biting and chewing. Instead of eliciting a phasic and continuous biting motion, touch of the gums may elicit a tonic and uncontrolled bite in infants with CNS dysfunction; release of the bite is often difficult.

The gag reflex is elicited by touching the posterior part of the tongue or palate. This protective reflex is present at birth. When the infant starts to chew on solids, the area sensitive to the gag reflex is gradually reduced and restricted to the posterior part of the oral cavity. In the neurologically impaired infant, the gag reflex is often hyperactive, especially in combination with swallowing problems. Absence of this protective reaction, also connected with CNS dysfunction, poses a hazard and needs to be considered when feeding the infant.

Breathing Patterns

Successful manipulation of food requires coordination between feeding and breathing, since the pharynx forms the passage for both food intake and respiration. Swallowing is alternative and dominant over respiration (Doty and Bosma). In the suckling infant, the rhythm of both breathing and swallowing is influenced and directed by the sucking center (Peiper). In the neurologically impaired infant, the interaction between sucking, breathing, and swallowing may be disorganized, which can lead to choking and aspiration.

The baby should be described as either a nose breather or mouth breather. In normal development, the infant must breathe through the nose up to three months of age. The infant with CNS deficit often relies on mouth breathing which increases the danger of swallowing air and aspiration. Since nasal respiration requires approximation between tongue and soft palate, a motor disturbance in these areas may contribute to patterns of abnormal breathing.

After reviewing and correlating the information gathered during the postural assessment, feeding, and oral examination, the therapist concludes the report with recommendations for appropriate intervention.

Appendix Motor Evaluation

Name: Chart no.:   Birth date: Date: Therapist:

I. General Impressions (alterness, interaction with parent/environment, communication, reaction to stimuli):

II. Sensory Deficits and Other Pertinent Medical Information:

III. Motor Functions

Motor Patterns:

Motor Functions	Normal Postural Adaptations	Abnormal Postural Responses	Postural Tonus

1. Observation of spontaneous behavior	1. Righting against gravity
	   extension
	   flexion
	   lateral flexion
	   axial rotation
		1. Exaggerated tonic reflexes
		   progravity pull into flexion/extension
		   obligatory asymmetry
		   pronounced adduction at hips
		   pronounced plantarflexion of ankle
		   fisting of hands
			Normal
			Hypotonic
			Hypertonic
			Rigid
			Fluctuating
			Associated reactions at rest
			change of tonus in response to stimulation, handling, movement

2. Elicit specific reactions if not displayed spontaneously:
   righting
   rolling
   transitions
   Landau reaction
   equilibrium
   protective extension
	2. Head control
	   face vertical
	   mouth horizontal
	   neck elongated
	   (after 4 mos.)
		2. Hyperestension of head and neck; lack of flexion against gravity (after 3 mos.)	

3. Test for mobility and postural tonus	3. Symmetry, midline control (after 4 mos.)	3. Persistent scapular protraction/retraction	
	4. Shoulder girdle (scapular) stability (after 4 mos.)	4. Total extension, pronounced/compensatory flexion	
	5. Differentiation and variation of movements		

Appendix (Continued)

Motor Functions	Motor Patterns: Normal Postural Adaptations	Abnormal Postural Responses	Postural Tonus
	6. Postural stability and mobility equilibrium reactions protective extension of arms (starting at 6 mos.)	5. Pronounced anterior/posterior pelvic tilt 6. Stereotyped patterns (frog position) 7. Paucity/excess of movement 8. Lack of mobility	
A. Prone Horizontal Suspension			
B. Supine, pull to sit			
C. Sitting			
D. All fours			

Appendix (Continued)

Motor Functions	Motor Patterns: Normal Postural Adaptations	Abnormal Postural Responses	Postural Tonus
E. Standing, vertical suspension			
F. Locomotion, gait			
G. Manipulation, eye–hand coordination, protective extension of arms			

IV. Overall Quality of Motor Behavior (variability, grading, sequencing):

V. Predominant Motor Patterns:

VI. Restricted Mobility, (Risk For) Contractures, Deformities:

VII. Reaction to Sensory Stimulation (kinesthetic, tactile, auditory, visual):

VIII. Additional Comments:

IX. Summary:

　　Displayed behaviors seem to be typical–, if not give apparent reason:

X. Program Goals:

IX. Recommended Procedures:

7
Home Management

The immediate environment of an infant is controlled and represented by the family who determines to a great extent whether the infant will reach full physical, intellectual, and emotional potentialities. The quality of stimuli provided by the family shapes early learning. Initially, babies depend mostly on their mother to provide these early learning situations through her attention while feeding and caring for them, playing and communicating with them. The success of the infant in achieving continued independence and control over actions and the environment, depends on how the parents relate and interact with the child.

While the infant's behavior is affected by the family, the family's behavior towards the infant is shaped by the infant's responses. Disturbed behavior resulting from central nervous system (CNS) dysfunction can inhibit interaction between infant and family. A baby's lack of responsiveness or irritable behavior is likely to decrease the family's desire to play and interact with him or her. When abnormal postural reactions make handling difficult, the infant may be held and cuddled infrequently. When the mother struggles to feed or bathe her infant, social interaction is likely to be omitted during these activities and feedback to the baby is scarce and negative. The baby with poor control of posture and movement is furthermore seldom encouraged to assist and participate to full capability, however limited, in activities of dressing and feeding. As a consequence, the child may become more and more passive and dependent, and lack of interaction deprives the handicapped infant of experiences normal babies are exposed to, which may further retard and disturb development.

In addition to receiving reduced handling and interaction, the infant with motor disturbances is often carried, dressed, fed, etc. in an abnormal fashion because the parent adapts to the baby's aberrant reactions. Through constant repetition, these abnormal reactions are reinforced and become, in time, firmly established, posing a severe obstacle to the learning of new and more complex skills.

The emotional impact on the family caused by severe delay and disturbance of development can be detrimental to both the infant and the family. Difficulties in meeting the most vital needs of a baby often cause severe frustration and anxiety in a parent; a feeling of inadequacy and even resentment may emerge. Appropriate counseling must attempt to alleviate such destructive reactions. Early intervention for home management should be a high priority in every infant program. The therapist must help parents to find the most efficient way of handling and caring for their infant. Parents must be educated and trained in how to behave appropriately so as to help reinforce and maximize the infant's skills while continuing to feel adequate in their own role as parents.

Advice in home management is tailored to the individual needs of each patient as well as his or her family. Instructions in specific handling techniques are most effective when they can be carried out in the patient's home. The parent who is taught basic concepts of normal and abnormal development and who understands general principles of intervention is better equipped to generalize handling techniques to accommodate a variety of situations. Parents should be taught which postures are conducive to different movements and which severely limit or inhibit motor activities. One way in which parents may learn about limitations of movements is to experience these limitations on themselves during training sessions.

Group sessions for parents are another way to present this information. The social aspect of parent groups is a further bonus of this type of parent training; the opportunity for sharing experiences and feelings with parents of other handicapped infants can be extremely valuable and supportive. Parent-infant sessions, on the other hand, are best carried out on an individual basis.

This chapter addresses home management on a general, conceptual basis, describes normal and abnormal postures which accompany motor functions of home management, and gives some samples of specific handling techniques. It does not include recommendations for fostering language, perceptual, and cognitive skills.

POSITIONING AND SEATING

A major concern of the management program is proper positioning and seating to allow the infant to function to optimal potential during play activities and feeding.

The family is faced with considerable problems in seating the severely impaired infant who lacks head and trunk control. The baby who lacks sufficient extension against gravity is not able to raise the head when prone and prop on elbows or hands. As a consequence, these infants usually spend the day lying supine. Without sufficient flexion against gravity this position is very restrictive and hypotonic as well as hypertonic infants are quite inactive when they lie straight on their back. Due to abnormal postural tonus, it is difficult or impossible to lift the head and/or raise the legs for any active body exploration and for investigation of the surroundings. Without control against gravity the infant cannot roll towards the side or towards prone but is locked into the supine position. If the shoulders are retracted, the child cannot bring the hands together preventing them or objects to reach the mouth for stimulation and investigation. Resulting limitations of sensorimotor experiences and reduced interaction with the environment contribute to perceptual impairment, delay of body awareness, disturbance of body image, and the problem of tactile hypersensitivity, especially in the oral area.

Better positioning becomes a high priority. However, it must be stressed that there is no one optimal or ideal position for the developmentally delayed infant. It is important to foster postural control in a *variety of positions*. The infant who cannot change positions without assistance, should be repositioned frequently and must be provided with optimal (not maximal) support in each position.

Supine Position

NORMAL DEVELOPMENT

Early play activities and initial manual and oral investigations take place in supine. Relatively high flexor tonus already affords the newborn some antigravity postures and movements in supine. More controlled and deliberate patterns of flexion, however, start to evolve at about three months of age when the baby assumes a more symmetrical posture with the head predominantly in midline position. This is a prerequisite for bringing hands together and for engaging in hand to feet, feet to mouth, and other exploratory activities. By five to six months, control against gravity in supine has progressed so that the baby is able to lift head unassisted. The primitive total patterns of flexion are gradually differentiated and are combined with components of extension and rotation providing the infant, finally, with the ability to move out of the supine position unassisted into sidelying, prone, or sitting.

ABNORMAL DEVELOPMENT

Abnormal postural tonus interferes with control against gravity and causes the infant to sink or to push into the support. Optimal positioning and support are required to foster proper control against gravity.

Normal and Abnormal motor patterns occurring in supine are described in detail in the section on "Postural Control in Supine," Chapter 4.

Positioning. Since turning the head to one side encourages extension, orientation of toys and other stimuli should stress midline position of the head when patterns of extension and asymmetry are predominant. Support of the head, shoulders, and upper trunk in a slightly flexed position allows the infant to bring arms forward and to keep the head in midline. Predominant extensor tonus can also be reduced when the pelvis is elevated and, thus, spine and hips are flexed. A ribbon or a bell fastened around the ankle draws attention to the legs and feet and stimulates flexion and midline orientation.

Equipment. A slightly flexed supine position can be achieved when wedges or pillows are placed under the head and/or pelvis. Flexion of hips and spine is also encouraged by propping the baby over an inflated tube, or by being placed in a hammock. Depending on the size of the netting, a lining may be required to prevent fingers or limbs from becoming entangled. Elevation of either end modifies the pattern and degree of flexion. Toys can be strung on stands or above the crib. Correct placement of the toys is essential for proper neck elongation and to enable the infant to reach them with the hands or to kick them with the feet. Frequently, toys are positioned directly above the head instead of further caudal as they should be to encourage neck elongation and tucking of the chin.

Prone Position

Babies develop independent postural control first in prone. This process is initiated with the development of head control, which in prone is achieved by four months of age. By five months, the infant can push up on both hands while prone. By six months, the infant has developed equilibrium reactions and between six to eight months, full extensor control is demonstrated in the Landau reaction.

The infant who demonstrates abnormal progravity extension in supine should be frequently positioned in prone in order to develop greater normal antigravity extension. The parent must be instructed in the correct postures which make lifting the head and propping on the arms possible. Normal and Abnormal motor patterns occurring in prone are described in detail in Chapter 4, section on "Postural Control in Prone."

Positioning. With the pelvis off the supporting surface, much of the body weight rests on the upper trunk which limits the degree to which the infant can raise the head. Hip extension is necessary to stabilize the pelvis on the supporting surface. When the legs are widely abducted as in the typical "frog" position, hip extension cannot take place. The legs must, therefore, be placed in a pattern of extension and slight abduction of the hips. If necessary, sandbags or bolsters are placed alongside the legs to maintain proper positioning.

During upper extremity weight bearing, scapular protraction and internal rotation of the shoulder can be reduced when elbows (or hands) are placed somewhat forward in relation to the shoulders. The parent is shown how to correct protraction and elevation of the scapula with one hand placed across clavicula, shoulder, and scapula while bringing the infant's arm forward with external rotation of the shoulder. Some support alongside the arms, for example, sandbags or bolsters, keeps the arms in proper position. Prone on elbows or hands is a very tiring position and is never maintained for long periods. The handicapped infant also should not be propped on elbows for an extended time. Instead, positioning in prone should make it possible for the infant to push up on hands or elbows when ready. Upper extremity weight bearing occurs also when the infant lies flat on the support with the shoulders fully flexed and the arms overhead. This position increases mobility between scapula and arm and is a good sensory preparation for upper extremity function.

Equipment. Placing the infant on an incline, such as provided by a foam wedge, may facilitate extension of the spine. For security and to facilitate hip extension, a restrainer can be used across the hips. The use of a roll or rolled towel to support and elevate the chest may cause the infant to pull the shoulders into extension and internal rotation against it which should be corrected.

Side Lying Position

The side lying position elicits lateral righting of head and trunk, and dissociation of motor patterns which leads to a pattern of overall extension on the weight-bearing side and a pattern of overall flexion on the non-weight-bearing side (amphibian reaction). This degree of postural control is achieved normally by 5 to 6 months. The infant with problems of postural control rarely assumes side lying. Nevertheless, the infant with dominant progravity flexion and/or extension probably has the best chance to move more normally and more effectively when lying on side.

Positioning. Proper postural alignment must be ensured. Undue extension must be corrected; the trunk should be straight or slightly flexed and not arched into extension; the head must be well-aligned with the trunk. Proper placement of toys encourages flexion of neck and head. A pillow under the head is used to facilitate lateral righting of the head and trunk. While the leg on the weight-bearing (lower) side is extended, the "upper" leg (on the non-weight-bearing side) is positioned in flexion. This facilitates differentiation of motor patterns. When necessary, a pillow separates the legs and maintains the flexed position. Where internal rotation of the non-weight-bearing hip is a concern, the flexed knee should rest on a small pillow. Both arms are brought forward and bimanual activities as well as interaction with toys is encouraged. The infant should, of course, be positioned on each side alternately.

Equipment. The infant who cannot remain in a side lying position, and rolls unintentionally and uncontrolledly towards supine or prone is supported by a bolster in the back. When more support is needed, a stuffed animal or a sandbag can be placed in front of the chest. For classroom use it is convenient to build a sidelying board that can be tilted into different angles from the horizontal.

Sitting Position

NORMAL DEVELOPMENT
The newborn attempts to align the head vertically in sitting, but, due to biomechanical and tonal conditions, the spine is flexed, so that the back is slightly and evenly rounded. A four-month-old infant can sit supported with fairly good head control. Although a six-month-old infant sits unsupported for brief moments, the sitting posture indicates that trunk control is not yet fully developed; increased adduction of the scapulae and "high guard" position of the arms compensate for the flexion of the lower part of the spine. By nine to ten months the trunk is stable during unsupported sitting, the back is straight, and the arms come down. Now, sitting balance is completed and the baby is able to pivot and to reach in all directions, although these activities may still produce traces of "high guard" posturing.

ABNORMAL DEVELOPMENT
The infant with developmental delay requires support for a considerably longer time and to a much greater degree. Nevertheless, the infant should not be deprived of the opportunity to view the environment from a sitting position. However, even when well-supported, the infant with poor head and/or trunk control who has not yet developed extension of the lumbar spine should only sit for short periods at a time. Normal and abnormal development are further described in detail in the section on "Postural Control in Sitting," Chapter 4.

Positioning. The following postural components should be applied regardless of which and how much support is given. The hips must be flexed sufficiently to have the infant sit square on the buttocks, which allows extension of the lumbar spine. Weight bearing must be symmetrical on both hips. The alignment between shoulders and the hips determines head and trunk posture; perpendicular alignment in the sagital plane requires good integration between flexion and extension. When the shoulders are forward of the hips, the infant has to use extension of upper trunk and neck to counteract gravity; when the shoulders are behind the hips, flexion is encouraged to overcome gravity. A slight degree of flexion, especially of the head, is desirable.

Equipment. A slightly reclined seat encourages the infant to lean against the back of the chair and tilt the head slightly forward. The angle between seat and back support is kept at ninety degrees. In order to achieve a straight back, the lumbar spine may require additional support.

The infant who shows a tendency to push into extension and to slide forward in the chair is ideally seated with hips and knees at a ninety degree angle. In this case, the depth of the seat must be adjusted so that the knees can be comfortably bent while the infant sits all the way back in the seat; when the seat is too deep, the hips can be pushed easily into extension. A padded back panel can be inserted to adjust the depth of a highchair. Elevation of the seat in the front encourages the infant to slide all the way back. A nonslippery surface also reduces the danger of sliding forward. When a seat belt is required for stabilizing the pelvis in a symmetrical position, it should be attached in a forty-five degree angle to the seat.

A laptray or table gives security and provides a base for toys. A lip around the tray prevents objects from sliding off. When the chair is reclined, the angle of the tray may have to be tilted too.

When head and trunk control are very poor, lateral support is attached to the back of the chair enveloping both shoulders and preventing retraction of the arms. Lateral support for hips and legs provides symmetry and prevents marked abduction of the hips. Triangle chairs are widely used when trunk control is poor; although they provide good lateral support, the support to the low back must be evaluated to ensure proper extension of the back.

The head position is extremely important and needs special consideration. Any tendency to hyperextend the neck should be discouraged. Adequate hip flexion and proper trunk extension are often sufficient for achieving a normal head posture. When additional head support is indicated, it should be shaped according to the form of the head; a straight extension of the back panel pushes the head too much into flexion in an upright chair and can be very uncomfortable. Footrests must be reached comfortably. The footrest for a reclined seat should be appropriately tilted to discourage pronounced plantarflexion.

For the infant with poor sitting balance it is often advisable to build a supportive seat insert which can be used in a highchair, chair and carseat. When such a seat insert is used exclusively, it should be made adjustable to provide a variety of sitting postures. Infant seats with adjustable seat depth and angle of recline and with lateral support to trunk and hips are available commercially.

Equipment such as baby swings and highchairs usually fail to provide postural stability: they often require specially designed attachments or inserts following the concepts described above. Poor posture is also displayed in baby jumpers and baby walkers, which are favorites for infants and parents because they provide the baby with some mobility. Parents must be made aware that "standing" and "walking" without proper support and consequently with poor postural alignment do not teach the baby how to balance. On the contrary, they aggravate abnormal tonus and postures throughout the body and may reinforce structural deformities of feet and hips. This equipment is widely advertised to be used at a very early age (four months), which is earlier than an infant's motor and structure ability will allow the child to stand for long periods of time.

Independent Sitting

The infant who sits independently may also need some monitoring of sitting posture. When sitting on the floor, the hypotonic infant often spreads the legs in wide abduction. This wide base poses little challenge for balancing and does not encourage movement and postural changes. Parents are advised to reposition the baby's legs and gradually decrease the degree of abduction. Placement of toys all around the baby elicits balance and protective reactions.

Sitting on the floor in "W" position (sitting between the heels) is frequently seen in handicapped children; it may be functional for a short time but it restricts the development of balance reactions and may lead to contractures when used excessively. Therefore, it should be replaced by other forms of positioning, as described above, or with supported sitting or sitting on a chair if independent longleg sitting cannot yet be achieved.

Car Safety Seats and Strollers

Principles described above also apply to the selection of car safety seats and strollers. Contoured seats with snuggly fitting lateral trunk supports work best when head and trunk control is a problem. Some carriages may only work after a supportive seat insert is attached. The umbrella stroller has found wide use for infants with a tendency to push into extension; however, the lack of a firm back support reinforces pronounced flexion of the lumbar spine and interferes with good trunk and head position. Strollers which are adapted specifically for the handicapped infant but can nevertheless be folded easily are commercially available; adaptations include trunk support, head support, and thigh separator.

With any model of car safety seat or stroller, a seat belt across the hips secures the infant in the seat; for this purpose the seat belt must cross the hips diagonally. Too often it is attached to the back panel instead of the seat and thus holds the infant across the abdomen which does not prevent him or her from sliding forwards underneath it. If additional support around the trunk is needed, a second belt can be added.

Standing with Support

NORMAL DEVELOPMENT
Supported standing seems to please babies at a very early age. The four-month-old may try to stand on feet when helped to a sitting position. The ability to pull to standing unassisted emerges during the last months of the first year when the baby commences to acquire balance in the upright position.

ABNORMAL DEVELOPMENT
The handicapped infant also enjoys the upright position but needs substantially more support and guidance to achieve correct postural alignment so as to develop a sense of balance.

Normal and abnormal patterns of standing are discussed in detail in the section on "Patterns of Standing" in Chapter 4.

Positioning. Standing balance can be encouraged while the child leans against a coffee table, couch or chair. It is important that the center of gravity is well aligned over the base of support. Frequently, help is needed to bring pelvis and hips far enough forward. Hip extension and upright posture is facilitated when the feet are placed very close to the furniture which is used for support. External rotation of hips and eversion of feet broaden the base and may increase stability but interfere with weight shifting and balancing. The infant should therefore also be encouraged to stand with the feet straight forward.

Equipment. Prone boards, which are available commercially, and supine boards are helpful for the infant who still cannot pull to a standing position during the second or third year. Their support can be adjusted for a wide range of balancing skills: as freestanding units or to be placed against a table or kitchen counter.

Standing tables and infant walkers are only support mechanisms and offer little possibility for selective correction of posture. Without correct postural alignment, standing may be more detrimental than helpful; abnormal postures resulting from poor support during standing may range from poor head posture to distorted foot alignment. Poor foot alignment and abnormal patterns of weight bearing often result in pronounced adduction, flexion, and internal

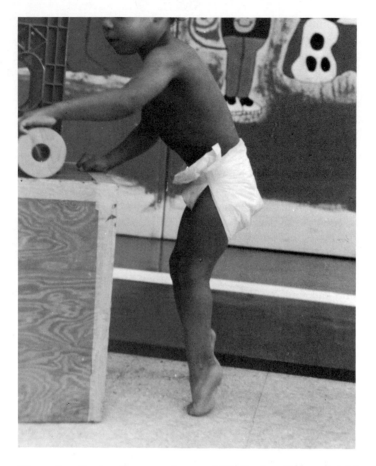

Figure 1a   During the second year of life the handicapped child enjoys
pulling to standing although he or she may lack the appropriate motor control. As a result, posture and tonus become increasingly abnormal.

rotation of the hips, which severely interfere with the development of standing balance. The effects of these postural maladjustments may, in time, also
be seen in other positions and may impair previously developed skills.

For proper alignment in standing, the hips must be brought into extension.
On the prone board hip extension is ensured with a belt across the hip joints
(Fig. 1a and b); when the hip belt is attached too high, the child sinks into
flexion. On the supine board a belt across the thighs and knees is often suf-

Figure 1b Placed on a prone board, good postural alignment and proper stability can be achieved with a belt across the hips. Rotation within the body axis and independent head movements are now made possible. Abnormal posture and tonus of the legs have been corrected. The closer the board is to the vertical position, the less demands are placed on righting head and trunk against gravity while lower extremity weight bearing increases.

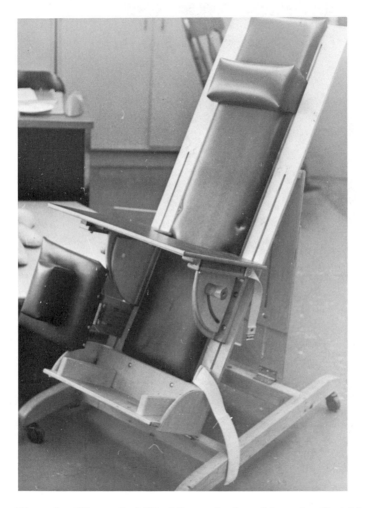

Figure 2a   The vertical tilt of the supine board is made adjustable. A slight backwards tilt encourages righting in the direction of flexion against gravity. A lap tray, adjustable in height and tilt, is used for security and for placement of toys. When indicated, a head support and a support across the thighs (not knees) can be attached.

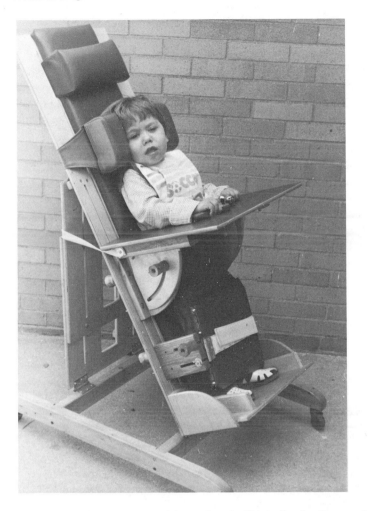

Figure 2b The supine board is used to facilitate the development of proper support tonus and righting against gravity in the vertical plane. A neutral posture of the pelvis allows proper hip extension and proper alignment of head in space.

ficient depending on the angle in which the board is reclined (see Fig. 2a and b). Otherwise, an additional belt is used across the lower rib cage. Foot placement determines the base of support; the hips should be slightly abducted and in slight external or neutral rotation. Some degree of hip abduction can be achieved with a wedge between the thighs. Pronounced external rotation or marked abduction result in weight bearing on the medial border of the foot.

Good weight distribution throughout the foot must be stressed and standing on the toes in plantarflexion is to be corrected. In case of structural foot deformities, the use of appropriate shoe inserts is indicated. If this option is not available, wedging of the footrest accomodates abnormal supination of the forefoot which can be a cause for excessive forefoot pronation in standing.

Lateral trunk support corrects asymmetrical trunk posture. The chest cushion and lateral trunk supports should not be too high, but should allow the infant to move the arms freely for propping and play activities.

The prone board facilitates extension against gravity while the supine board encourages the infant to counteract gravity by slightly flexing neck and upper trunk. The incline of the board determines the degree of antigravity activity which decreases progressively for upper trunk and head the closer the board is to the vertical position. As with all equipment, the prone and supine board should be used only for brief periods. The infant's position should be changed frequently. This is especially important for the severely disabled patient where the therapist has found one good position (after many attempts).

CARRYING

NORMAL DEVELOPMENT
During the first weeks of life a baby seems to struggle with balancing a relatively oversized head, succeeding only momentarily in attempts to hold the head upright while placed against a mother's supporting shoulder. In the second month, however, the infant can prevent severe head drops when being carried. By four months, good head righting and some trunk righting responses are established and parents report that the baby feels "firm and put together." The parent adjusts spontaneously by withdrawing total support of head and trunk.

ABNORMAL DEVELOPMENT
The infant with disturbed motor development requires prolonged postural support and is, therefore, held and carried in a more infantile, frequently reclined, position which gives little opportunity to right the head and trunk. The baby who is carried in a more upright position is often held with no regard to the shoulder girdle posture. Attempts to align head and trunk without a stable shoulder girdle posture result mostly in the head flopping from too much flexion to too much extension. Lack of shoulder girdle stability leads to shoulder elevation, which presents a poor base for proper head righting. When lifting, parents tend to hold around the thorax and lift in a suspended supine position. The infant with motor difficulties is not able to

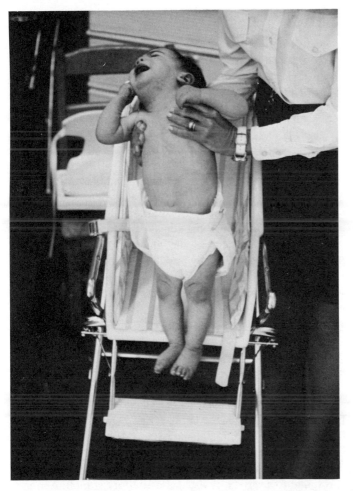

Figure 3a Hyperextension of head and neck may result when the infant is held in a suspended position while supported only around the thorax. The accompanying extensor hypertonicity makes it very difficult for the infant to sit in a highchair (from *The Infant with Cerebral Palsy: An Approach to Identification, Management and Treatment*, A. L. Scherzer. Private printing, New York, 1973).

align head and trunk (Fig. 3a). The head falls back or is pulled into extension. The whole body may stiffen in response to the abnormal head posture which makes it very difficult to place the infant in a highchair or bathtub. The parent who carries the baby on the shoulder and always on the same side may reinforce an existing asymmetry of trunk and pelvis.

To cope with the numerous problems posed by poor head and trunk control, some parents place the infant into a baby carrier which is strapped around the parent's shoulders with the baby either in front or in back. The support provided by most baby carriers is not firm enough; the baby then sinks into too much flexion of the spine and consequently has to hyperextend the neck to lift the head. These infant carriers seem to be a poor imitation of an Indian custom where the baby is tightly wrapped in a long shawl which then is wrapped in many different ways around the mother's shoulders and trunk. The tight wrapping provides stability and maintains a close contact with the mother's body.

Handling. The infant experiences more normal righting and balancing when given proper support. It makes sense to take advantage of the fact that, during carrying, the parent's movements cause a continuous shift of the baby's center of gravity, therefore eliciting postural adjustments and readjustments. Principles for proper postural alignment are the same as those for seating and are therefore, only briefly outlined. A more upright position makes head and trunk righting easier. In addition to the orientation in space, the alignment between shoulder and pelvic girdle also determines the degree of extension or flexion of the spine (see "Positioning and Seating, Sitting Position"). Trunk balance is inhibited and the posture of the shoulder girdle impaired when the infant "hooks" one arm around mother's shoulder. Asymmetry of the pelvis leads to asymmetry of trunk and head.

1. The infant faces the parent who places one arm across the infant's back and holds one or both thighs, with the hip(s) flexed. The baby may sit on the parent's hipbone. Some trunk rotation and slight flexion of head and upper trunk is facilitated from the pelvis. Trunk support should be sufficient to make the infant feel secure but minimal enough to provide opportunity for normal balance reactions. Depending on the degree of head and trunk control, the infant turns head and trunk in response to the surroundings and in this position can respond to a variety of visual and auditory stimuli. Abnormal arm and shoulder girdle postures, such as retraction, must be corrected.

2. The same upright position is maintained but the infant faces away from the parent (Fig. 3b). According to the degree of head and trunk control, the baby leans more or less against the parent's body. Both arms are brought forward and confined between body and arm of the parent when retraction of the arms is a problem. The degree of hip extension is changeable as well as the extent to which the spine is extended or flexed; in the case of predominant extensor patterns, the trunk is slightly reclined. A component of trunk rotation can be introduced.

3. When it is not possible to correct abnormal retraction of arms with the above method, the parent is advised to hold the baby facing away while

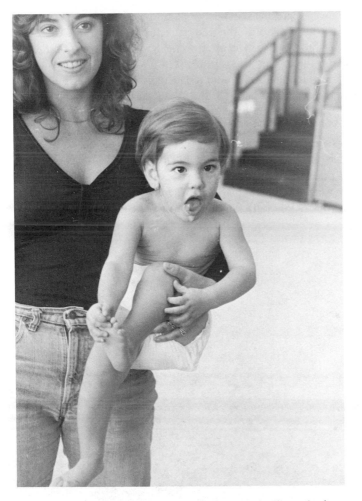

Figure 3b More appropriate head righting is facilitated when one or both hips are flexed while the infant is carried in an upright position. Free observation of the surroundings and reaching can occur. Note the rotation within the body axis.

holding each leg, keeping the hips in flexion. In this position, the parent's arms are then placed firmly against the baby's arms, preventing their retraction.

4. The arms can also be brought forward and over the parent's shoulder when the baby is held against the parent's shoulder and supported across the back.

5. Instead of always carrying the baby in an upright position, the parent may occasionally tilt the child onto the side to elicit dynamic lateral righting and amphibian reactions (Fig. 4). The infant is held around the arm on the lower (weight-bearing) side. This arm is brought into external rotation and complete abduction which facilitates unilateral elongation of neck and trunk. The parent places the other arm between the infant's legs and holds the baby either around the trunk and chest or, if the infant displays a strong tendency towards shoulder retraction, around the other arm. When winging of the scapula is a problem, the parent can support the scapula on the elongated side instead of placing the hand on the infant's chest. The baby's head may rest on the abducted arm or on the parent's arm. When more support is needed, the infant's back rests against the parent's body. When lateral righting does not occur spontaneously, caudal traction is applied form the arm on the flexed

Figure 4 Occasionally, the infant may be tilted on his side when carried. Good posture of the shoulder girdle is achieved when the weight-bearing arm is supported in an externally rotated position. Lateral righting of head and trunk must be encouraged (photograph by Carol Herwig).

(upper) side. Postural adjustments can be varied by deviating from the horizontal plane or by tilting the infant partially toward supine or prone.

6. Complete prone position can be chosen for facilitation of extension against gravity. Again, the infant can be carried either in a completely horizontal or a more upright plane. The mother supports the infant under both externally rotated arms and places her other hand between the baby's legs to support the chest and abdomen from underneath.

Lifting. Difficulties of head righting are especially obvious when the infant is picked up from the supine position. Rather than lifting the baby in a suspended supine position, the parent is instructed to roll the baby partially towards one side which offers a better position for active flexion of neck and head. When lifting the infant out of the highchair or stroller, the parent places one arm across the baby's back, tilting the child's head and trunk slightly forward while supporting and holding both thighs with one or both hands.

BATHING

The difficulties of handling the developmentally impaired baby increase during bathing because the baby's wet body becomes extremely slippery. The baby's and the parent's insecurity and tension may turn a basically joyful activity into one colored by apprehension.

Before placing the infant into the tub, the parent must carry and hold the baby in the most symmetrical and normal posture with proper alignment of head and trunk and adequate hip flexion. The tub should be equipped with a nonslip surface for better stability. When sufficient postural control cannot be provided by the parent, a commercially available bath seat is recommended, secured against sliding with suction cups or suspended from the rim of the tub. A child's swimming tub or a plastic clothes basket also provide some support and can be equipped with a seat belt if needed. Bathing in a small tub or in the kitchen sink makes it also easier for the mother to handle the infant who has poor postural control.

A floating toy or one tied to a string in front of the infant encourages proper head position and adds to the pleasure of taking a bath. It may be helpful to wrap the baby in a towel before being taken out of the tub.

DRESSING

NORMAL DEVELOPMENT
Toward the end of their first year, babies start to participate actively in undressing and dressing. By that time they have learned that the arm goes through the sleeve; they hold out their feet to have shoes put on, or try to

pull off their socks. By about eighteen months to two years of age they can help in undressing but still need help in dressing for some time.

ABNORMAL DEVELOPMENT

The infant with CNS deficit shows considerable delay in dressing abilities. Some children may always need substantial help, but too often they are kept in a totally passive role. When sitting balance is impaired, the infant is usually dressed while lying flat on the back and cannot see and observe the parent while being dressed. Consequently, the child never learns how to participate.

Dressing Situation

Dressing is an activity where much learning can take place. Names of body parts and different clothing or actions, spatial relationships, laterality, crossing of midline, and sequencing of activities (socks before shoes) are some of the concepts which can be stressed during dressing. Balancing, weight shifting, and propping are motor reactions which occur naturally. Communication between the parent and the infant is an important aspect of this activity as of all activities of caretaking; the parent must be made aware of continuing the communication even though the infant may not be able to answer.

Positions For Dressing

SUPINE

Flexion against gravity can be facilitated when the infant is dressed in the supine position. The pelvis is elevated which makes it possible for the infant to watch how pants, socks, and shoes are put on or taken off. With some encouragement the baby may reach towards the feet and help more or less with the chore. Rotation between shoulders and pelvis can be easily incorporated and stressed during this activity and may lead to rolling. Rolling the baby from side to side is necessary when the shirt is to be put on in this position. Dressing in supine can be carried out on the dressing table but also very comfortably on the parent's lap (Fig. 5).

SITTING

The infant who has achieved some trunk control is seated on the dressing table and dressed from the front. This is an excellent time to practice and improve sitting balance, because the center of gravity is continuously shifted. Propping on the hands is encouraged initially while the parent lifts the baby's foot and leg to put on socks, shoes, and pants. Later, the baby may be able to balance while pushing the limbs or head through garment openings. Gradually, the infant participates more in the activity, for example, pulling off a

Figure 5 When the infant is dressed on the parent's lap, proper flexion of head and hips can be facilitated by elevating the pelvis in the supine position. Correction of scapular retraction permits the infant to reach forward and participate in the activity. Rotation within the body axis can easily be incorporated (photograph by Marion Madigan).

sock after the parent has pulled it halfway down over the heel. The baby who cannot participate on this level is guided from shoulder or arm.

The infant who is less independent in sitting is dressed with the parent providing support from behind. Sitting on the parent's lap during dressing allows even more control of trunk and arm movements. In addition, weight shifting can be accentuated when the mother moves her legs. Trunk rotation and guidance from shoulder or arm are used to facilitate reaching (Fig. 6).

SIDE LYING
In the side lying position the baby is also able to observe dressing activities. The infant who is hypertonic while lying face upwards may be reasonably relaxed when turned side ways and thus may be able to stretch arms forward to reach garments and touch legs. To encourage lateral righting and proper head position, the head should be supported on a small pillow or folded towel.

Figure 6   Sitting balance is provided with support from behind. The posture of the left leg decreases extensor spasticity and reinforces more dissociated leg movements. When seated upright and securely supported, the infant can observe and participate in undressing and dressing.

PRONE

Dressing in prone is especially suited for babies with a strong tendency to push into extension. It is best carried out with the infant lying on the parent's lap, where sweaters and shirts can easily be pulled off in a backwards to forwards motion. This facilitates flexion of the neck while removing a garment front to backwards over the head may reinforce extension. Lateral weight shift and trunk rotation can be practiced during dressing. The parent should be instructed to support the infant well under the stomach if the infant has a tendency to sway back. Caution is also indicated when the infant tends to pull into flexion from the arms. Instead of having the arms hang over the parent's leg they should be brought forward into full overhead flexion and some external rotation while weight bearing occurs on the long side of the arms. This position cannot be used to encourage self-dressing, but can be beneficial for the parent of a stiff baby.

Handling Principles

The parent needs further advice on specific handling principles to improve and facilitate dressing. Care should be taken not to elicit a stretch reflex by pulling on the infant's hand while trying to get an arm through a sleeve. An increase of flexor tonus may be the response to this pull and hamper cooperation. It is much easier to straighten the arm by pushing the elbow forwards and upwards. The parent of a hemiplegic or very asymmetrically impaired infant is advised to put the garments on the more affected limbs first. Specific handling techniques are also required for putting on shoes when the infant plantarflexes the ankles tightly and curls the toes. These difficulties are reduced when the leg is brought into flexion and foot and toes are dorsiflexed. Unlacing and opening the shoes completely makes it possible to control and correct the position of foot and toes in the shoe. Once the toes are dorsiflexed they can be held in this position by pulling back on the infant's sock near the toes. If the infant pulls the heel up, the parent provides downward pressure from the flexed knee before lacing the shoe.

Clothes

The right choice of clothes plays some part in reducing the difficulties in dressing. To put on a tight turtleneck or overall outfit may require extensive stretching and twisting of the limbs and can leave both the infant and the parent frustrated. It is much easier to pull arms through garments with the opening and fastenings in the back. Large openings and clothes that can be stretched reduce the necessity for moving limbs in complicated and difficult patterns. However, foot coverings of elastic material can reinforce clawing of the toes and should not be pulled too tight.

MOBILITY

During the second half of the first year a baby develops different and increasingly more effective forms of locomotion. The infant with CNS impairment, on the other hand, is very restricted in mode of progression and may use excessive extensor patterns while pushing along in supine, or excessive flexor tonus may result from pulling forwards in prone. The reinforcement of asymmetrical postures is also a concern during locomotion. The more severely impaired infant may experience considerable frustration at not being able to move around without assistance.

It is therefore no surprise when both infant and parent are delighted to realize that a baby walker provides this mobility. As discussed earlier in this chapter under the section "Standing with Support," the disadvantages in most cases outweigh the advantages of such a walker. Other means of providing mobility should be found.

Equipment

A well-adapted scooterborad is one possibility. It allows the infant to push around in prone while being supported in a well-aligned posture. The hips are a very important point of control and are to be stabilized in extension with a strap. Undue adduction of the hips can be prevented by a wedge between the thighs. Proper trunk extension can be facilitated by slanting the front of the board upwards. Shoulder blocks may be helpful for trunk symmetry and for preventing retraction of the arms.

As with most equipment, scooterboards are widely overused and are not always sufficiently adjusted to the individual patient. Without good support, some infants demonstrate increased spasticity and/or abnormal movement patterns as a result of the effort and excitement involved. The quality of such learning experiences is certainly questionable.

Mobility equipment to be used in sitting by the older infant and by the toddler include different types of "toddler riders" and, later on, tricycles. They require a thoughtful design. Pelvis and trunk must be stabilized to allow for the necessary mobility of the limbs. Applicable concepts have been discussed in the section on "Positioning and Seating." When internal rotation and adduction of the hips need modification, a wedge is placed between both thighs. Scapular protraction and internal rotation of the shoulders can be neutralized when the handlebars are brought into a vertical instead of horizontal position.

FEEDING

Difficulties in feeding the infant with CNS deficit may seriously interfere with a family's daily routine. Impaired oral development often results in unacceptably long feeding sessions, and can cause considerable frustration and anxiety for infant and parent.

Immediate intervention is necessary to interrupt and reduce these adverse influences and is of primary concern where malnutrition is possible. Appropriate feeding management helps also to counteract the development of abnormal and possibly grotesque feeding patterns which may keep patients dependent for the rest of their lives, limiting social integration and acceptance. The specific information obtained during the oral evaluation and the recommendations emerging from this assessment constitute the basis of a feeding program. This program has to consider all factors influencing abnormal oral behavior.

Positioning

Posture and position accompanying feeding should be considered first. The head position in particular is decisive for the distribution of tonus and greatly influences oral posture and function. Infants are often fed in a reclined position when sitting balance is impaired and when food cannot be transferred back by the tongue (Fig. 7a). A child kept in this disadvantageous posture

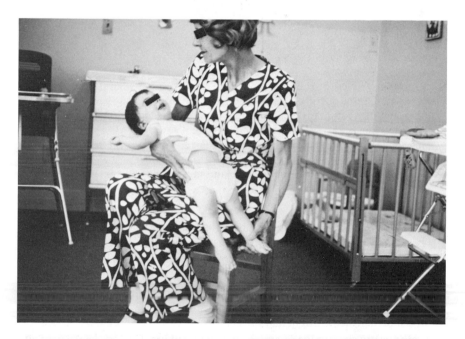

Figure 7a Extensor spasticity is aggravated when the infant is held in the supine position. Head and arms are pulled back and the back arches which makes it very difficult to support and balance a baby. In addition, this position puts severe limitations on the infant's active interaction with the environment (from *The Infant with Cerebral Palsy: An Approach to Identification, Management and Treatment*, A. L. Scherzer. Private printing, New York, 1973).

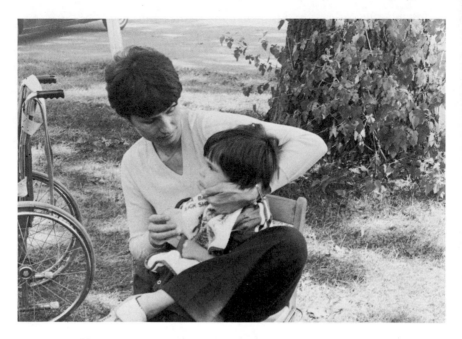

Figure 7b   When the infant is fed seated on the parent's lap it is important to stress an upright posture of head and trunk. Support to the low and mid-back may be required to achieve some degree of head flexion. The parent's knee can be used to support the child's back. "Jaw control" also corrects any tendency to head retraction or turning and tilting of the head. The arms are brought forward for proper posture of the shoulder girdle. The grasp around the jaw monitors oral posture and movement (see text).

cannot develop active manipulation of the food and will always rely on the assistance of gravity for swallowing. It is therefore imperative to select a position as upright and symmetrical as possible. Providing sufficient postural support and good stability makes the task easier for everybody involved. Improving the infant's position may result in spontaneous improvement of vegetative functions. Optimal feeding patterns seem to be linked to optimal positioning in the patient with CNS deficit.

By five to six months of age the normal baby has developed sufficient sitting balance to be fed while sitting in the highchair. When possible, the developmentally impaired infant should also be fed sitting in a highchair or seat insert. Guidelines for the design of corrective and supportive seating arrangements have been discussed previously. See section on "Positioning and Seating, Sitting Position."

The same concepts for postural control apply to the infant who is fed on the parent's lap. Appropriate hip flexion can be obtained by having the baby's buttocks slide down between the parent's legs (Fig. 7b). Placing one foot on a stool helps the parent to increase the amount of the infant's hip flexion, or, with the other leg, to support the baby's back against the knee, while resting the arm on the knee or on a nearby table. It is important that the seating arrangement be comfortable for the infant and the parent otherwise it will deteriorate during the feeding session.

Another feeding position has been described by Helen Mueller. She places the infant with poor head control on a wedge or pillow in a semireclined position. Sufficient flexion of the head and hips counteracts abnormal extensor patterns. For this arrangement, the infant sits on the parent's lap facing the parent; a wedge or pillow is placed behind the child's head and back while leaning against the edge of a table.

James Bosma recommends feeding the child with swallowing problems in prone. Proper positioning in prone and on the prone board has been described previously (see "Standing with Support"). It should again be stressed that sufficient extension against gravity is necessary for adequate head control in prone. The severely hypotonic infant may raise the head with excessive extensor tonus or may rest too heavily on the chin when given "jaw control" (see the section on "Jaw Control"). This can lead to abnormally high tonus in the oral area. Positioning on the prone board in a more upright position diminishes these problems.

In addition to the infant's position, attention should be given to the parent's position in relation to the infant. Placement of the food and how the parent approaches the infant also influence head position. Too much head extension, for example, is encouraged if the food is presented from above. To correct hyperextension of the neck and reinforce midline orientation the food should be presented from the front.

Jaw Control

Although appropriate positioning greatly improves oral function, further control of oral responses may be indicated for the severely impaired patient. This specific control can be achieved with a facial grasp or "jaw control." By placing one finger under the chin directly behind the mandibular bone, mouth closure can be reinforced. Extension and retraction of the mandible can also be inhibited with this control. Placing one finger in the depression between chin and lips can initiate opening of the mouth and inhibit mandibular protrusion. Lip closure can be facilitated by gently pushing upward along the lower lip. Attention must be paid not to provide too much pressure to this sensitive area. A very light touch is also extremely stimulating and may also adversely affect tonus. Caution should be exercised so as not to push the head into hyperextension while facilitating jaw closure. When this grasp around the chin is not sufficient to control mandibular deviation, the palm of the hand or the index finger is placed along the side of the mandible. Proper head flexion and midline orientation can be obtained by manipulating the head with the described grasp around the chin. For additional inhibition of hyperextension of the neck, some pressure is applied to the sternum with the lateral portion of the hand or with the long side of the little finger.

The facial grasp can be applied from the side and from the front (see Fig. 7b). In general, the side grasp allows more control over the head position, because the parent's arm behind the infant's head together with the grasp around the chin prevent the infant from pushing the head back. The parent will need some practice and occasional supervision by the therapist to become efficient in these techniques. A common error is to pull the chin too far forwards which results in hyperextension of the neck. The head position should then be corrected by pushing the chin towards the chest while providing jaw closure. Attention is also necessary so as not to pull the mandible to one side, nor to turn the head laterally. As the infant gains more control over the oral mechanism, the use of the facial grasp is no longer required and should be gradually discontinued. After establishing sufficient control of posture and oral responses the infant is prepared for food intake.

Feeding Procedures

To facilitate normal feeding patterns and inhibit abnormal feeding responses, the therapist must have a thorough knowledge of oral development. Both normal and abnormal feeding patterns as well as underlying components and subskills have been described in the section of feeding evaluation (see Chap. 5.)

Sucking. Sucking at the breast is easier for the infant with CNS impairment if held in a more upright position or when placed on one side. Extensor patterns should be corrected, especially retraction of shoulders, arms, and head. Some support under the chin (jaw control) may improve the efficiency of the suck–swallow pattern.

The success of bottle drinking depends to a great part on the proper selection of the nipple. A nipple which is too long for the infant's mouth hinders proper tongue movements. A nipple with a big opening allows free and constant flowing of the liquid into the mouth which the infant will not be able to regulate through the sucking action. The abundance of liquid is a particular problem for the infant with swallowing difficulties. The therapist, therefore, should personally test the nipple by tilting the bottle upside down. There should be no free and constant flow of liquid. A short round nipple with a small opening is the proper choice. The use of a "bottle straw" which can be attached to any nipple allows the infant to empty the bottle without tilting the head back and is very helpful for feeding the handicapped infant. The consistency, taste, and temperature of the liquid chosen may also influence sucking patterns. Responses to different qualities of liquids are described in the following section.

Cup Drinking. The normal infant initiates cup drinking by the age of five to six months. The infant with feeding difficulties is usually fed by bottle for much longer. When cup drinking is finally initiated the baby is frequently given a spouted cup which encourages the child to retain primitive or abnormal sucking patterns. The handicapped infant is thus not given a fair chance to develop more mature feeding habits. The exaggerated licking action of the tongue and lack of lip movements yield very inefficient drinking patterns, especially for cup drinking. Early initiation of cup drinking under proper guidance helps to counteract the habituation of poor feeding patterns and is an important step in fostering more normal development.

The application of the facial grasp helps to reduce a predominant suck; the jaw is stabilized, lingual and mandibular movements decrease, and more discrete lip movements are facilitated. Furthermore, sipping movements are stimulated by the sensory input of the liquid touching the lips. This requires that the cup be not placed too far into the mouth. Placing the cup on the teeth or biting surface does not encourage sipping, but reinforces sucking and biting. It must be remembered that the aim is to have the infant take the liquid in with the lips and not the tongue. Jaw and lip closure must also be facilitated during swallowing.

It is particularly difficult for the handicapped baby to manipulate thin and watery liquids. Slightly thickened liquids provide a stronger stimulus for labial sipping movements and are easier to gather into a bolus for swallowing. Creamed soups, melted ice cream, nectars, loose puddings, and milk shakes are some of the liquids to be chosen. Gradually, liquids of thinner consistency are included in the diet. Taste and temperature need consideration. Sweet substances reinforce sucking. Taste can also affect the flow of saliva: some fruits, such as apple, lemon, and orange stimulate increased salivation, as does chocolate. These liquids should not be given to infants with severe swallowing difficulties. Extreme temperatures often elicit hypertonicity in the oral area.

Another consideration is size and material of the cup. A small cup can be emptied more easily than a large one, without having to tilt the head too far back. The cup should be made of a pliable, durable material, especially for the infant with an obligatory bite reflex. Breakable plastic cups must be avoided. The pliability of a cup allows the parent to form a spout to reduce spilling when the infant cannot yet sip efficiently. Helen Mueller suggests cutting a notch out of the rim to allow room for the nose and make it possible to empty the cup without tilting the head too far back. It also helps the parent to monitor the flow of liquid.

Spoon Feeding.   Many mothers introduce one or two spoonful of solids by
the time the baby is about 3 months old, which is shortly after the infant
learns to swallow voluntarily. The five- or six-month-old baby is eating solids
for a substantial part of his or her diet. The switch from sucking to effective
handling of solids is, of course, gradual. Initial attempts at spoonfeeding are
not very successful because the infant uses sucking motions. Spoonfeeding
the infant who has not only primitive feeding reflexes but also abnormal
sucking and abnormal swallowing patterns is therefore a greater challenge.

In order to monitor abnormal sucking and swallowing patterns, jaw control is essential. The exaggerated opening of the mouth which is one component of an abnormal suck has to be inhibited. Jaw control modifies and weak-
ens exaggerated tongue motions and an obligatory suck. To inhibit the forward thrusting of the tongue further, downward pressure on the tongue can
be applied with the spoon. This accentuated sensory input may also prompt
proper action of the lips for taking the food off the spoon. The spoon should
not be put too far into the mouth and should be removed quickly before the
baby bites down on it. It should always be held horizontally. Care must be
taken not to tilt the spoon nor scrape it along the teeth since this may result
in retraction of the lips. Assistance for jaw and lip closure is to be continued
until swallowing has occurred. The upper lip should not be pulled down passively because the hypersensitive infant reacts to this with spasticity. Lip
closure and protrusion of the lips are elicited more successfully from the lower lip or the corner of the mouth.

Proper selection of the food contributes to the success of spoon feeding.
As with cup drinking, thinner consistencies are difficult to control and aggravate drooling. Mixed consistencies, such as vegetable soups and some prepared baby food dinners should not be presented to the infant with impaired
oral perception and disturbed coordination. It requires special skill to sort
and manipulate different consistencies. Foods such as mashed potatoes,
cooked cereals, or puddings are recommended for initial attempts at spoon
feeding. Most foods can be prepared in the baby strainer without liquifying
them. Increasing the repertoire of textures, tastes, and temperatures is a long-
term goal of this program.

Shape, size, and material of the spoon must be taken into account. For
safety reasons, plastic utensils should be excluded. Teflon-coated or rubber-
tipped spoons are helpful for infants with a strong bite response. The depth
of the spoon's bowl affects lip activity and must be adjusted to the infant's
capabilities. A flat metal spoon, such as the "mother care" spoon makes re-
moval of the food easier. A spoon with a very small, narrow bowl which can
be placed on the tongue without hitting the lingual sides of the teeth is effective for feeding the infant with a strong bite reflex.

Biting and Chewing.   As a first step in teaching the patient how to manipulate solids, he or she must be assisted in the inhibition of the suck and bite re-

flexes. Jaw control suppresses extreme depression of the mandible and allows chewing or munching movements. The jaw should not be moved passively in a rotary motion so as not to interfere with the coordination between movements of lips, tongue, and jaw. Introducing the food from the side and placing it directly on the chewing surface discourages sucking and facilitates tongue lateralization. It may be necessary initially not only to place the food on the biting surface but also to hold it there during the infant's attempts at chewing. This will influence the selection of food.

As with drinking and spoon feeding, the type of food presented to the infant can drastically affect success or failure. Baby foods, sandwiches, and peanut butter and jelly encourage sucking. Crackers are too dry and tend to scatter, making it difficult to form a bolus. Crusts and hard bread, dried fruits, hard cheese, cooked vegetables, and strips of meat are recommended textures. Taste and temperature again must be considered.

The nutritional value of food is especially important for the infant with severe feeding problems and the advice of a dietrician is strongly recommended. Frequent and short feeding sessions may work best when feeding problems are serious.

Self-Feeding. Infants begin to finger-feed at five to six months of age and handle utensils with moderate spilling by about two years of age. The handicapped child may never achieve total independence, but should nevertheless, be encouraged to participate as actively as possible. Otherwise, total dependence on others for feeding can pose emotional and social problems later. Appropriate support, assistance, and specific adaptations may be required.

An infant can only finger-feed or handle utensils when seated securely without the need of hands for support. Guidelines for seating have been given in the preceding section "Positioning and Seating, Sitting Position".

The selection of food should follow the above recommendations.

When utensils are used, their safety has to be considered. Plastic should not be used. The infant who tightly fists hands when grasping should be given a spoon with a built-up handle in order to widen the grasp. The parent may teach self-feeding effectively stabilizing the spoon with thumb against the infant's palm. The parent's fingers at the dorsum of the infant's hand guide the infant's hand movements. Taking the food off the plate may be as challenging as bringing the food into the mouth. The food is easily pushed off the plate or the plate slides away. A plate with a high curved rim is very helpful and can be further stabilized by being placed on a nonskid pad.

The hand not being used for feeding should be placed on the table to diminish associated reactions and ensure trunk symmetry. This is especially important for the hemiplegic child.

It is important not to overlook oral reactions when teaching the infant how to manipulate different feeding utensils. The effort used in self-feeding can elicit abnormal oral tonus and associated reactions in the oral area. In order to reduce this abnormal sensory feedback, it is recommended that the infant's hand be guided and jaw control is provided until independence in the most normal fashion is achieved.

ORAL HYGIENE

Oral hygiene is of special importance in the infant with feeding problems, since the restricted diet and lack of intrinsic tongue movements do not help to clean teeth, gums, and palate. Without proper oral care, gums deteriorate, especially in the infant who is on anticonvulsive medication.

Even before teeth erupt, the gums should be cleaned after each feeding with a moist towel wrapped around the parent's finger. This can also be used for oral stimulation, adapted to the baby's level of tolerance, while controlling motor responses with proper techniques of jaw control. In the hypersensitive infant, very light touch elicits very strong reactions, and the parent should be careful not to elicit a gag reflex.

Later on, a small, soft toothbrush is introduced and rinsing of the mouth is carried out with warm water. In order to facilitate spitting, head flexion is important and the infant can be further assisted with gentle forward pressure towards the cheeks.

With this feeding program, the infant will, it is hoped, soon be able properly to manage a healthy diet conducive to dental and oral health.

SUMMARY

The infant with sensorimotor deficit is often handled in a way that encourages primitive and passive behavior. When the parent adjusts to the infant's abnormal postural reactions, abnormal postures and movements are established and become habitual. Reinforcement of primitive and abnormal behavior aggravates developmental delay.

Intervention in form of specific handling methods has been described in this chapter and designed to interrupt abnormal sensorimotor behavior while fostering more normal development. The handicapped infant is able to participate actively in dressing and feeding when placed in more advantageous positions and provided with corrective, proximal support. When well-positioned and securely seated, the child can manipulate and investigate toys. With appropriate guidance, the parent gains skill and confidence in handling the infant who lacks adequate postural control. The parent also learns to foster the infant's independence.

To optimize the patient's potential and encourage the development of mature patterns of posture and movement it is necessary to provide more specific handling and more selective stimulation through a well-designed treatment program.

APPENDIX Infant Management Evaluation

Name: Birth date: Chart no.:
Diagnosis: Date: Examiner:

I. General Impressions (family situation, daily routine, activities and habits, availability and appropriateness of toys):

II. Functional Abilities and Areas of Strength (head control, trunk control, manipulative skills, ability to adjust to handling, awareness, social/ physical interaction, grasp patterns, eye-hand coordination):

III. Areas of Major Difficulties:

IV. Carrying, Lifting:
1. Present procedures (postural adaptations, active participation by infant, approach by parent, tolerance towards handling):

2. Postural Reactions Interfering with Proper Adaptations to Being Carried:

poor head control	_____	pronounced flexion of lumbar
poor shoulder girdle		spine _____
stability	_____	one/both arms retracted _____
asymmetry (head,		excessive, uncontrolled
spine, pelvis)	_____	movements _____
others:	_____	poor tolerance towards
		handling _____

3. Risk for Development of Contractures, Deformities:

4. Postural Corrections and Support Needed for Optimal Function:

hip flexion	_____	trunk rotation _____
back support (lumbar)	_____	hands to midline _____
trunk vertical, pelvis		extended posture (prone) _____
level	_____	hips abducted _____
others.	_____	

5. Summary:

6. Recommendations:

V.   Positioning:
1.   Present Procedures

2.   Evaluation of Postural Adaptations and Functional Abilities:
      Supine
a.   Spontaneous Postures, Motor Functions, Postural Tonus:

b.   Postural Corrections and Support Provided: Functional Abilities:

head flexed	pelvis elevated	shoulder support		
_____	_____	_____	hands to midline, symmetry	_____
_____	_____	_____	goal directed reach, play	_____
_____	_____	_____	changes position	_____
_____	_____	_____	equilibrium reactions	_____

      Prone
a.   Spontaneous Postures, Motor Functions, Postural Tonus:

b.   Postural Corrections and Support Provided   Functional Abilities:

hips extended	pelvis stabilized	on incline		
_____	_____	_____	free head movements, neck elongated	_____
_____	_____	_____	leans on elbows	_____
_____	_____	_____	hands	_____
_____	_____	_____	reaches for toys	_____
_____	_____	_____	changes position	_____
_____	_____	_____	equilibrium reactions	_____

      Sidelying
a.   Spontaneous Postures, Motor Functions, Postural Tonus:

b.   Postural Corrections and Support Provided: Functional Abilities:

head elevated	trunk supported (back,	front)		
_____	_____	_____	hands to midline, plays	_____
_____	_____	_____	changes position	_____
_____			equilibrium reactions	_____

Sitting: on floor; in highchair, chair; on parent's lap
a. Spontaneous Postures, Motor Functions, Postural Tonus:

b. Postural Corrections and Support Provided: Functional Abilities

hip flexion 90°	lumbar spine supported	back vertical	back reclined	knees flexed		
					symmetry (head, trunk,	
_____	_____	_____	_____	_____	pelvis	_____
_____	_____	_____	_____	_____	head control, neck	
_____	_____	_____	_____	_____	elongation	_____
_____	_____	_____	_____	_____	leans on hands	_____
_____	_____	_____	_____	_____	hands free for play	_____
_____	_____	_____	_____	_____	equilibrium reactions	_____
_____	_____	_____	_____	_____	changes positions	_____

3. Summary:

4. Recommendations:
Positioning, Postural Alignment:

Equipment:

Adaptations to highchair, stroller, mobility equipment:

VI. Dressing
1. Present Procedures (postural adaptations and active participation by infant, approach by parent, type of clothing):

2. Postural Reactions Interfering with Dressing:

poor sitting balance	_____	excessive uncontrolled	
thrust into extension	_____	movements	_____
pull into flexion	_____	tight flexion of arms, fisted	
others:	_____	hands	_____
		tight adduction of hips	_____
		plantar flexed ankles, curled toes	_____

3. Positioning and Handling Procedures for Optimal Function:

Supine:	pelvis elevated	_____	incorporating trunk rotation	_____
	flexion of head	_____	pushing arms through sleeves	
Sitting:	trunk support	_____	(no pull)	_____
	hip flexion	_____	flexing hips, knees	_____
Prone		_____	ankles, toes dorsiflexed	_____
Sidelying		_____	others	_____

4. Summary:

5. Recommendations:
   Positioning:

   Handling:

   Clothes:

VII. Feeding
1. Present Procedures:
   Positioning (infant's posture, approach by parent, equipment):

   Oral posture, tonus, movements (jaws, lips, tongue);

   at rest:

   during sucking:

   during spoon feeding:

   during biting, chewing:

   during self-feeding:

2. Factors Interfering with Food Intake:

   Posture:

   Approach by parent:

   Selection of food, utensils:

   Abnormal oral tonus, abnormal oral sensitivity:

Primitive/abnormal oral reflexes:
rooting _____ suck–swallow _____ phasic bite _____
tonic bite _____ hyperactive gag _____ hypoactive gag _____

Structural deformities:

Teething:

Respiratory problems:

Choking, vomiting:

3. Intervention and Its Effect on Feeding.

Positioning:
upright position of head, trunk:

head slightly flexed:

support to lumbar spine:

prone position:

sidelying:

Selection of food as to consistency, taste, temperature, texture:

Selection of utensils:
nipple size, size of opening:

rigid straw:

size and shape of cup:

size and shape of spoon:

Handling:
jaw control:

approach from front:

spoon held horizontally:

food placed on biting surface:

guidance for self-feeding:

4. Summary:

5. Recommendations:

Positioning:

Handling:

Food, Utensils:

VIII. Bathing
1. Present Procedures (postural adaptations, active participation by infant, approach by parent, equipment):

2. Postural Reactions Interfering with Bathing:

poor head control	_____	hypotonic ("frog") posture	_____
poor trunk control	_____	excessive, uncontrolled	
thrust into extension	_____	movements	_____
pronounced flexion	_____	others:	_____

3. Postural Corrections and Support Needed for Optimal Function:

head supported in flexion	_____	midline orientation, symmetry	_____
hips flexed	_____	hands to midline	_____
neutral hip abduction	_____	others:	_____

4. Summary:

5. Recommendations:

Positioning:

Handling:

Equipment:

IX. Postural Tonus
normal _____ hypotonic _____ hypertonic _____ rigid _____
fluctuating _____
Change of tonus with stimulation, handling, movement:

X. Sensitivity (kinesthetic, tactile, auditory, visual stimuli):

XI. Factors Interfering with Daily Care

abnormal extensor tonus	_____	poor head control, poor righting	_____
abnormal flexor tonus	_____	poor balance and proximal	
lack of support tonus	_____	stability	_____
postural asymmetry	_____	hypersensitivity towards	
lack of mobility	_____	handling	_____
		unresponsiveness	_____
		others:	_____

XII. Risk for Developing Contractures, Deformities:

XIII. Additional Remarks:

XIV. Summary

Displayed behavior seems to be typical _____, if not give apparent reason:

BIBLIOGRAPHY

Ardran, G. M., Kemp, F. H., and Lind, J.: A cineradiographic study of bottle feeding, *Br. J. Radiol.* 31:11, 1958.

Ardran, G. M., Kemp, F. H., and Lind, J.: A cineradiographic study of breast feeding. *Br. J. Radiol.* 31:154, 1958.

Ardran, G. M., Kemp, F. H.: Some important factors in the assessment of oro-pharyngeal function. *Dev. Med. Child Neurol.* 12:158–166, 1970.

Bobath, B.: The very early treatment of cerebral palsy. *Dev. Med. Child Neurol.* 9:373-390, 1967.

Bosma, J. F.: Human infant oral function. In Bosma, J. (ed.): Symposium on Oral Sensation and Perception. Springfield, Ill., Chas. C Thomas, pp. 98-111, 1967.

Bosma, J. F.: Physiology of the mouth, pharynx and esophagus. In Otolaryngology. Philadelphia, Saunders, pp. 356-370, 1973.

Bosma, J. F. (ed.): Fourth Symposium On Oral Sensation And Perception. Washington, D.C., U.S. Government Printing Office, 1973.

Bosma, J. F., and Showacre, J. (eds.): Development Of Upper Respiratory Anatomy And Function. (Symposiom). Washington, D.C., U.S. Government Printing Office, 1975.

Doty, R. W., Bosma, J. F.: An electromyographic analysis of reflex deglutition. *J. Neurophysiol.* 19:44-60, 1956).

Finnie, N. R.: Handling The Young Cerebral Palsied Child At Home (2nd ed). New York, Dutton, 1975.

Hochleitner, M.: Betreuung des cerebral bewegungsgestörten Säuglings (Handling), Mutteranleitung. Göttingen, Institut für den Wissenschaftlichen Film, Medizin 4, 12, C 1241, 1978.

Illingworth, R. S.: Sucking And Swallowing difficulties in infancy: diagnostic problems of dysphagia. *Arch. Dis. Child.* 44:238, 1969.

Ingram, T. T. S.: Clinical significance of the infantile feeding reflexes. *Dev. Med. Child Neurol.* 4:159-169, 1962.

Morris, S. E.: Program Guidelines For Children With Feeding Problems. Edison, N.J., Childcraft Educational Corp., 1977.

Mueller, H. A.: Facilitating feeding and pre-speech. In Pearson, P. H., and Williams, C. E. (eds): Physical Therapy Services in the Developmental Disabilities. Springfield, Ill., Chas. C Thomas, pp. 283-310, 1972.

Mueller, H. A.: Feeding. In Finnie, N. (ed).: Handling the Young Cerebral Palsied Child at Home. New York, Dutton, 1975.

Sameroff, A. J.: Reflexive and operant aspects of sucking behavior in early infancy. In Bosma, J. F. (ed.): Fourth Symposium on Oral Sensation and Perception. Washington, D.C., U.S. Government Printing Office, pp. 135-151, 1973.

Straub, J.: Malfunction of the tongue: Abnormal swallowing, its cause, effects and results in relation to orthodontic treatment and speech therapy. *Am. J. Orthod.* 46:404-424, 1960.

Davis, L. F.: Pre-speech. In Connor, P., Williamson, G., and Siep, J. (eds): Program Guide for Infants and Toddlers with Neuromotor and other Developmental Disabilities. New York, Teachers College Press, pp. 183-205, 1979.

Wilder, C. N.: Respiratory Patterns In Infants: Birth To Eight Months Of Age. Unpublished doctoral dissertation. New York, Teachers College, Columbia University, 1972.

Willoughby, M., Tscharnuter, I., and Fabricant, P.: Treatment Approaches To The Oral Developmental Needs In Cerebral Palsy. Instructional course lecture, American Academy for Cerebral Palsy, 1974, 1975, 1976.

Wilson, J. M.: Physical therapy and infant home management programs. Proceedings from The Comprehensive Management of Infants at Risk for CNS Deficit, May 1974. Chapel Hill, Division of Physical Therapy, University of North Carolina, Chapel Hill, 1975.

Wilson, J. M. (ed.): Oral Motor Function And Dysfunction In Children. Proceedings, May 1977. Chapel Hill, N. C., Division of Physical Therapy, University of North Carolina, Chapel Hill, 1978.

8
Treatment

Treatment of the infant with symptoms of cerebral palsy and related sensorimotor deficits cannot be restricted to the patient but must include the
family. Family involvement in handling the infant should go beyond intervention methods of home management discussed in Chapter 7 to include treatment procedures. When the parent carries out a home therapy program, the
infant is guided and assisted in development on a daily basis and within a
daily routine.

The therapist must nevertheless help the parent to put the home management and therapy program into the right perspective so as not to disturb the
parent–child relationship. Focusing the attention exclusively on the infant's
disabilities hampers rather than fosters overall development. Abnormal motor
patterns can be overemphasized. It is only the continuous repetition of these
patterns which interferes with normal development. The parent—and the
therapist—must understand that there are moments where therapeutic intervention must be secondary.

Instructions given to the parent must be thorough and detailed enough to
assure the quality of the home program. Handling techniques must be adapted to the skills of the parent and may consequently differ from the techniques the therapist applies to the same activity.

Good parent training ensures not only an intensive, continuous treatment program for the infant but frees the therapist to serve more patients. In accordance with this concept the therapist's role is not only to administer a treatment remedy but also, to a great extent, to act as advisor for the family.

NEURODEVELOPMENTAL APPROACH

Coordination of Movement Patterns

A major concept of this treatment approach is based on the conclusion that a lesion of the central nervous system (CNS) results in a loss of movement and not in a paresis of muscles [1]. Furthermore, it is believed that new motor skills are learned by learning "movement patterns and not a sequence of a mosaic of activation of specific muscles" [2]. Stretching and strengthening of individual muscles are consequently not considered to be therapeutic. Instead, a much broader approach must be chosen. In learning new motor skills, the focus is mainly on the coordination of movement patterns and their accompanying postures.

Relation Between Movement, Posture, and Postural Tonus

Normal movement patterns are accompanied by postures which are changing and therefore dynamic [3]. Postures also preceed and facilitate movement (some of these postures have been described in Chap. 7). The infant with a restricted repertoire of postures is limited in purposeful movements.

Both normal postures and normal movements are only possible with normal strength and distribution of postural tonus, while abnormal postural tonus is always combined with abnormal postures and abnormal movements. In therapy, the close interplay between movement, posture, and tonus is utilized. Modification of any one of these functions changes the others. For example, tonus can be changed by correcting abnormal postural alignment which, in turn, makes possible more normal movement patterns.

Automatic and Voluntary Movements

Another concept implies that proper adaptation of posture and tonus, and maintenance of balance are normally regulated by subcortical centers. Postural adaptations are mostly automatic, freeing higher cortical centers for planning intentional motor acts and a variety of mental and learning processes.

Patterns of voluntary movements are based on automatic postural reactions, such as righting, equilibrium, and other protective reactions [4] as well as on primary motor patterns which emerge in utero [5].

The goal of therapy is to elicit appropriate automatic reactions in response to handling. Working on an automatic level has the additional advantage of diminishing the increasing hypertonicity often resulting from the effort and anticipation involved in a remeditated act. The fact that motor responses can be elicited on an automatic level makes this approach largely independent of the patient's cooperation and level of mental function. Its application is therefore well-suited to the young infant.

Active Participation

The learning of new motor skills requires that they be carried out actively. It is not sufficient to maneuver the infant through different motor patterns while passive. An activity can be active even when assistance and support are provided, but this assistance must be kept at an optimal level to ensure active participation of the infant without eliciting an abnormal response as a result of stress and effort.

Automatic motor responses, such as righting and equilibrium reactions, although elicited on a subconscious level are as active as voluntary motions.

Interplay Between Various Motor Patterns

In normal development, primary motor patterns as primitive reflexes and early righting reactions, become increasingly complex or fade out as more mature automatic responses, such as equilibrium reactions emerge. In cerebral palsy, primitive reflexes, for example, tonic reflexes in time gain increasing dominance.

Persistence of primitive reflexes or poorly integrated motor patterns form a poor neurological as well as biomechanical base for the development of more complex motor skills. These early deviant motor components have been described as "blocks" which can be correlated with subsequent abnormal patterns as they develop caudally and distally [6].*

Facilitation and Inhibition of Postural Responses
Through Controlled Sensory Input

In treatment, the goal is to dampen (inhibit) abnormal postural reactions while fostering (facilitating) more normal and more efficient reactions, such as righting and equilibrium reactions. This is achieved by handling the infant and guiding his or her movements. Through handling, the therapist controls the sensory input to some degree and, in an indirect way, the motor output.

---

*Quinton, M. B.: Course in Neurodevelopmental Treatment Approach. Unpublished lecture notes, Seattle, Washington, 1978.

This results in a more normal sensory feedback which enhances the establishment of normal automatic responses and the subsequent learning of effective voluntary movements without the need to drill these skills.

Inhibition of abnormal motor patterns and facilitation of more normal patterns as an automatic response to specific handling techniques was first described by Berta and Karel Bobath [7] as the fundamental concept of the neurodevelopmental treatment (NDT) approach. Mary Quinton [8] has adapted these principles specifically to very early treatment, e.g., intervention within the first nine to twelve months of life.

GENERAL TREATMENT PRINCIPLES

Modification of Body Schema

Quality of motor behavior and learning of new motor skills depend on previous sensorimotor experiences and their internal representation, e.g., the body schema. The body schema is shaped and continuously reshaped by sensorimotor experiences. Modification of abnormal motor behavior can, therefore, be achieved by modifying and improving the patient's body schema through selective sensory input which indirectly controls the motor output and determines type and quality of sensory feedback. This sensory feedback should reflect purposeful sensorimotor experiences.

It seems that sensory preparation in the form of mobile weight bearing on different body parts precedes their respective motor control. For example, the infant rests most of the body weight on head and upper trunk in prone and supine before developing control of head and shoulder girdle. Treatment should provide similar sensory preparations.

Grading of Stimulation

The therapist's goal of providing as much normal feedback as possible must never result in a bombardment of multiple and diverse stimuli. A systematic approach is recommended with room for ample repetition of appropriate postural responses in a variety of positions and situations. Nevertheless, the intervention program must still strive for a balance of multiple motor patterns. Exclusive reinforcement of one motor pattern over a longer period of time contrasts with the sequence of normal development and may have adverse effects.

The selective and graded support provided, permits the therapist to bring the infant into a variety of positions even when the infant has only minimal postural control. Depending on the support given, the demands placed on the infant's balancing skills can vary widely in any one position. For example,

the infant with poor sitting balance can already be treated in supported standing as long as the therapist can provide proper postural alignment. Here, it
should be pointed out that parents place their babies into various positions,
such as supported standing, at a very early age and usually long before the infant achieves the respective developmental milestone.

Components of Movement

The treatment plan reflects the sequence of normal development. Complex
and skillful activities are based on a combination of simpler movement components acquired at an earlier stage of development. These motor components may be seen as "subskills," some of which econmpass the activities described in this chapter (see section on Specific Treatment Procedures). The
therapist should provide a solid foundation of these early and basic subskills
before working on more difficult motor tasks. Some of the most important
basic skills are righting of head and trunk, and proximal stability of trunk,
shoulder, and pelvic girdle. These require modification of primitive and total
motor patterns.

Although functional activities are a major concern, this approach puts
little stress on practicing these functional activities or developmental milestones per se. Instead it aims to provide the infant with the postural building
blocks required for a variety of automatic and volitional activities. A well-
founded knowledge of normal development allows the therapist to select
subskills required for activities of current as well as future developmental
skills and motor functions.

Dynamic Versus Static Treatment

Since the facilitation of righting and equilibrium reactions is one of the major
treatment goals, it follows that treatment must not be static but should
always be dynamic. Every movement is prepared and combined with weight
shift. Weight shift facilitates movement and can be used as a tool to elicit the
desired postural reactions. A small amplitude of weight shift is often used to
facilitate control of every phase of the activity.

The same approach is used when trying to increase mobility and achieve
elongation of muscles. Passive stretch and forceful resistance are not used. Instead, motor responses are facilitated which themselves result in active elongation. The same process can be seen in normal development, for example, in
the infant who rocks from side to side in the supine position with legs and
pelvis raised off the support which results in elongation of the extensors.
Through small range movements and weight shifting the infant is prevented
from building up abnormal tonus which would resist movement in the desired
direction.

Individualized Programs

The therapist must be aware of the impact that therapeutic handling has on the shaping of early sensorimotor experiences and the resulting body schema, the very tools upon which later skills will be based. The motor patterns which the therapist facilitates must, therefore, be as accurate and normal as possible. The need for thorough knowledge of normal developement and normal movement cannot be overemphasized. Relatively small deviations from the norm may prove to be limiting factors in highly complex skills as they develop during later developmental stages. Instructions to parents must be precise and detailed to prevent abnormal compensations.

The implementation of the program and the application of handling techniques must also take into account individual differences. Reactions to stimuli and responses to various aspects of handling vary considerably, depending for example on basic postural tonus. A play activity causing too much excitement and subsequent hypertonicity in one infant may not arouse another at all. Tempo and rhythm of movements influence tonus. Very slow and rhythmical movements allow the hypotonic infant to stabilize with habitual patterns of abnormal fixing and to fall from one end position into the other. Very fast movements, on the other hand, do not provide sufficient time for postural adjustments in the hypertonic infant. Orientation towards gravity affects postural tonus. With the hypotonic infant who sinks into gravity and who almost melts to the support, postural tonus may improve drastically in more upright positions. Given little support, these infants are forced to be more active while the baby with predominantly high tonus tightens up even more when feeling insecure. Amplitude of movements is another factor to take into account. Postural control must be achieved in a small range before full balance can be expected during large range movements.

Specific techniques of sensory stimulation such as approximation (cocontraction), tapping, vibration, etc., can change tonus drastically and need to be applied with good judgement. From the result of the evaluation, the therapist can predict to some degree the infant's reactions and can adjust handling appropriately.

Shaping Motor Behavior Through Handling

This approach uses "hands on" to elicit and shape motor responses. Touch in itself is, of course, a stimulus and appropriate grading must be adjusted to the individual. Very light touch is most stimulating and may cause withdrawal. A firm touch is preferable and is also more directive. It is, however, important not to provide undue pressure. It is not necessary nor desirable to embrace a patient with a tight grip. An open grip with extended fingers provides sufficient support and directive guidance. It also causes the pressure to be applied through the palm and/or long side of the fingers and prevents irritating localized pressure through the fingertips. In order to facilitate fine graded responses, the sensory input provided through the therapist's hands must be finely tuned and dynamic, i.e., using variation of pressure through the various parts of the hand.

A bombardment of tactile input caused by frequent changes of hand placement can be very disorganizing and overwhelming for a sensitive infant. When the therapist distributes sensory cuing all over the baby's body by jumping from one contact point to another, the infant receives confusing messages and may consequently react with irritation and crying—and with reason. A constant and firm contact from very few points of control (key points) is desirable and seems most effective.

The therapist handles the infant not just for support but to provide guidance (facilitation) and correction (inhibition) of postural reactions. The point of control must therefore be carefully selected. Proximal points of control, i.e., trunk, shoulder, or pelvic girdle permit the greatest impact on the motor patterns. Distal control is chosen as soon as the infant is capable of taking over a major part of postural control. The goal is of course to fade out the control provided by therapist or parent.

The amount of support and control is also adjusted to the individual infant. During balance activities the therapist should try to handle the infant mostly from the non-weight-bearing side to facilitate righting against gravity, while too much support on the weight-bearing side may encourage the infant to lean into gravity.

SPECIFIC TREATMENT PROCEDURES

Treatment procedures are categorized according to motor functions and their major components rather than by diagnosis. The motor functions are described in order of increasing degrees of complexity.

In every activity the main focus is on postural alignment (integration of righting reactions), control (function of equilibrium reactions), and the quality of individual movement components. Handling is described in detail to stress the importance of correct alignment and control. The techniques themselves are changeable and must be adapted to individual needs of patient, therapist, and parent. The selection of activities is limited and does not represent a complete treatment program. A concept for treatment and not a procedural outline is described here.

Some of the ideas underlying the following activities and handling techniques have been presented and generated during a neurodevelopmental training (NDT) course given by Mary Quinton and Elizabeth Köng in Seattle, Washington, June 19 to August 25, 1978, and during an NDT baby course presented by Mary Quinton in Roosevelt, New York, June 8 to 26, 1981.

HEAD CONTROL

Early signs of abnormality may occur in patterns of head posture. Even the baby who manages to lift and balance the head may do so in an abnormal or immature fashion. Without good head control, more complex motor functions and, indeed, learning about the self and the world is impeded.

Different degrees of head control and some typical abnormal compensations have been described in Chapter 4.

Righting Into Flexion Against Gravity

Fine graded postural adjustments of head and trunk require a delicate balance between axial flexion and extension. When this balance is impaired, shoulder girdle and trunk cannot provide a stable base for the head to move upon. Midline control and lateral righting are consequently difficult. Elongation of the neck cannot take place. Instead, tightness in the neck and shoulder girdle area may lead to contractures.

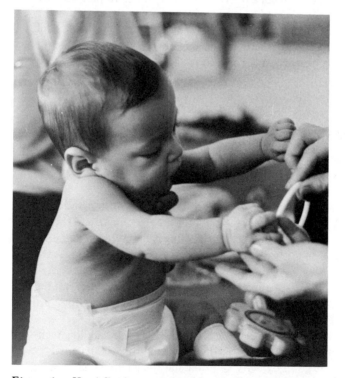

Figure 1a Head flexion and shoulder girdle stability are severely impaired and cause the head to tilt slightly back and to one side while the shoulders are extremely elevated (photograph by Marion Madigan).

Activity

Start at a point where good posture and balance of the head is easy to achieve; such as upright sitting. Facing the therapist, the infant is tilted slowly back; the goal is to elicit proper alignment between head and trunk. When the center of gravity is shifted behind the base of support, the pelvis tilts posteriorly and the spine flexes evenly. At a certain point of recline, the baby may elevate and flex the legs as a balance reaction.

Handling

To correct the shoulder position, the therapist holds the infant around the shoulders while pulling gently downwards and outwards. Instead of moving tho infant ropoatodly throughout tho whole range of the movement, the therapist rocks the baby gently in small lateral and anterior/posterior excursions. When the head falls back into extension, the infant is brought into a more up-

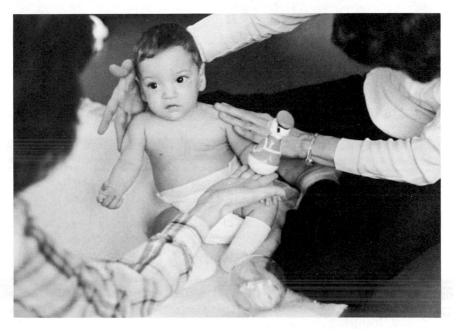

Figure 1b By stabilizing the shoulder girdle with a downwards/outwards pull, the therapist can facilitate flexor control against gravity while tilting the infant back in sitting. In order to shift the weight to one side, increased pressure is applied to the opposite shoulder in a diagonal direction; this facilitates lateral righting against gravity. Some downward pressure may also have to be maintained on the weight-bearing side to prevent improper shoulder elevation (photograph by Marion Madigan).

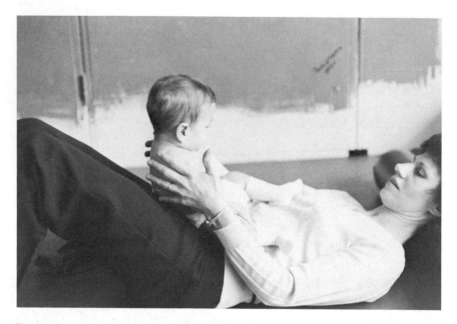

Figure 1c Neck elongation and head flexion can be encouraged by directing the infant's visual gaze accordingly. In this position, weight shifting and lateral righting can be induced through lateral movements of the therapist or parent (photograph by Marion Madigan).

right position. Pressure should be distributed on the shoulders in as broad an area as possible, because the shoulders are very sensitive to sharp and pointed pressure. Therefore, the fingers of the therapist or parent should be kept extended to prevent localized pressure from the fingertips (Figs. 1a and b).

Variations. Flexor control and neck elongation are further reinforced when toys are placed in front of the infant, or when the therapist or parent lies on back with the infant straddled across the lap (Fig. 1c). In this position, weight shifting and lateral righting reactions (see below) can be induced through lateral weight shift of the therapist or parent.

Midline Orientation

Flexor control leads to midline orientation and bimanual activities, such as hand to hand, mouth, knees or feet motion, or reaching for toys. Grasping and sucking may result in too much tonus (tightness around shoulder girdle), in which case the infant should be encouraged only to reach, swipe at, or hit objects.

Activity

Toys or other stimuli are presented in midline while the infant is in supported sitting as described in the section "Righting Into Flexion Against Gravity," or in a modified supine position, i.e., with the pelvis elevated and the spine straight.

Handling

Techniques of handling are described under activities in the section "Righting Into Flexion Against Gravity."

Lateral Head Righting

Lateral righting is an extremely important reaction which deserves high priority in the treatment of motor disabilities. It represents a major step beyond total flexion/extension and leads to rotation within the body axis which is an essential subskill for mature balance reactions. Some onset of lateral righting is obvious at an early stage of development (three to four months). In treatment, early facilitation of lateral righting helps to prevent the infant becoming locked into total and abnormal motor patterns.

Activity

The above activities are slightly modified. Instead of reclining the baby from sitting in a straight plane, lateral rocking and weight shifting are induced. The baby is rocked gently from side to side while tilted back. The amplitude of the lateral displacement must be adjusted to the infant's ability and may be very small at the beginning. With more lateral displacement, the trunk gradually rotates towards the non-weight-bearing side: the shoulder on the weight-bearing side is slightly forward in relation to the other shoulder. The infant who uses predominantly patterns of extension tends to rotate the trunk in the opposite direction. Proper frontal alignment between shoulder girdle and pelvis must be kept: the shoulder girdle should not be pulled sideways in relation to the pelvis.

Lateral righting combines lateral flexion towards the non-weight-bearing side with active elongation on the weight-bearing side.

Handling

From the non-weight-bearing side, the therapist elicits lateral flexion with downward traction through shoulder and arm. To achieve proper support tonus on the weight-bearing side, elongation of the trunk is facilitated. Care should be taken not to elevate the shoulder (see Figs. 1b and c).

Neck Elongation

Lack of mobility in the neck and shoulder girdle area interferes with refined head control.

Activities

Supine. The infant lies on the back with the pelvis elevated and the spine straight. The parent holds the infant around the shoulders and rocks the child gently from side to side while gradually increasing cervical flexion and elongation of the neck.

Handling

Both shoulders are pulled downwards and outwards and both arms are kept forward between the parent's arms to prevent the infant from pulling back shoulder girdle or arms. Optimal correction of scapular protraction can be

Figure 2a In supine, elevation of the pelvis is used to increase cervical flexion and elongation of the neck. This provides the infant with the sensory feedback of proper head alignment. Elevation of shoulders and scapular protraction must be corrected by handling the infant either from the shoulders while the pelvis is supported on the parent's lap or by applying traction from the arms.

achieved when the shoulders are pushed backwards with the parent's index finger or thumb. This also allows to accentuate the sensory feedback of weight bearing on the upper trunk and shoulder girdle area which is an experience the infant with abnormal postural tonus is often lacking. The pelvis is supported by the parent's body. The more the pelvis is elevated, the more the body weight rests on the upper trunk and shoulders and the more the stretch is applied to the back of the neck (Fig. 2a).

Sidelying. Neck elongation and dissociation between head and trunk movements can also be carried out in the sidelying position over a roll.

Handling

While holding the infant around the trunk, the therapist rolls the infant slightly towards supine, then back to sidelying and slightly towards prone. Care is necessary to prevent too much extension of the neck and retraction of the head (Fig. 2b).

Figure 2b Neck elongation and dissociation between head and trunk movements can also be carried out in sidelying position over a roll. By elevating the pelvis in relation to the shoulder girdle, the body weight rests on the shoulder which can be used to achieve depression of the shoulder girdle. The strong sensory feedback on the shoulder reinforces the experience of this postural alignment (photograph by Carol Herwig).

Body Righting Reaction on Head

This ensures proper postural alignment and enables the baby to roll, for example, from supine towards the side or towards prone. Predominant extension and asymmetrical tonic neck reflex (ATNR)-posturing as well as severe hypotonicity may suppress the reaction.

Activities

The baby is placed in supine position with pelvis and legs elevated to encourage flexion against gravity. Body righting reaction on head is facilitated by rolling the pelvis towards either side. As a reaction, the baby rolls trunk and head toward the same side.

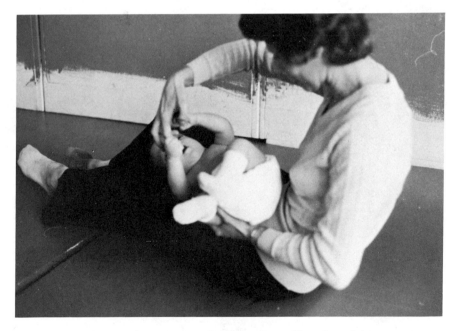

Figure 3a   Body righting on head is facilitated by rolling the pelvis to one side. Proper postural alignment between head and shoulder girdle must be maintained. When turning the head too far, pronounced extension may occur and must be corrected. Elevation of the pelvis inhibits excessive extensor tonus (photograph by Marion Madigan).

Handling

Scapular retraction and hyperextension of shoulders are inhibited (Fig. 3a). Elevation of the shoulder girdle must be corrected as described in the section "Neck Elongation".

Carry Over. In order to reinforce flexion against gravity, the parent is advised to use the above position frequently for dressing. Some degree of rotation between shoulder girdle and pelvis may evolve when, for example, removing or putting on pants. This rotation prepares body righting reaction on body (Fig. 3b).

To make active head flexion possible, the baby should be rolled halfway to the side when pulled to a sitting position or being reclined to supine. Control is provided through arms or shoulder girdle as required.

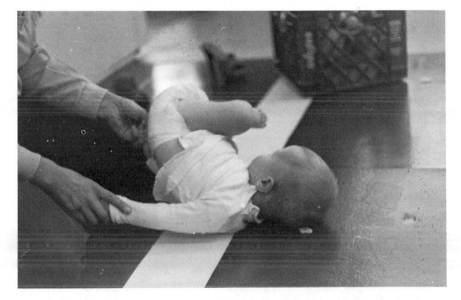

Figure 3b Body righting reaction on body is facilitated by rolling the pelvis to either side while controlling the posture of arms and shoulder girdle from the hands to achieve rotation within body axis (photograph by Carol Herwig).

TRUNK CONTROL

The development of head control overlaps the subsequent development of
trunk control. Free head movements are only possible with some stability of
shoulder girdle and trunk. Also, head movements elicit compensatory movements of the trunk. In supine, the neck righting reaction causes the baby
to roll to the side when the head is turned. The neck righting reaction is already present in the newborn and is well-developed by four months of age.
In prone, head and trunk move initially toward the side the baby turns to;
later on, as equilibrium develops, the body weight is shifted toward the opposite side which enables the infant to lift the non-weight-bearing hand and
reach towards objects in his or her field of vision. Intrinsic trunk movements
as required for righting and balance reactions are first prepared in supine and
in prone. Abnormal postural tonus and poorly integrated head control im-
pede further development of trunk control.

Integration Between Flexion and
Extension in Prone

When the baby raises the head in prone or prone propping, a flexor component ensures elongation of the neck. Assistance may be required to achieve this
mature posture of head and trunk.

Activity

The baby leans on elbows or hands in the prone position. The therapist observes that the elbows are slightly forward in relation to the shoulders to promote some degree of external rotation of the shoulders. The shoulders are
only slightly abducted so that lateral weight shift can take place. When visual
stimuli are used to obtain head righting reactions, they should be placed low
to elicit some degree of head flexion.

Handling

The therapist applies postural control from the shoulders to inhibit scapular
elevation and internal rotation of the shoulders. The palm of the therapist's
hands envelop the infant's shoulders. For more abdominal action, slight pressure is given at the chest with extended fingers. Lateral weight shift through
the trunk can be achieved when more pressure is provided to one shoulder in
a diagonal direction.

Variation. When more flexor control is required, the therapist supports the
infant under the abdomen or chest with extended fingers toward the infant's
shoulders for further control.

Integration Between Flexion and Extension in Supine

Integration between flexion and extension enables the baby to keep the head in midline with good neck elongation, to extend the arms forward and to grasp knees or feet, and so forth. Initially, the knees are flexed due to the tendency towards total flexor patterns. Only when differentiation of movement patterns is possible, can the infant combine flexion of the hips with extension of the knees. With hands on knees or feet, the baby rocks from side to side which demonstrates highly developed abdominal control and is a direct preparation for sitting balance. This degree of abdominal action and control is often omitted in the handicapped infant and results in lack of mobility and lack of movement differentiation between hip, pelvis, and trunk.

Activity

As noted in the activities for Neck Elongation and Body Righting on Head, the infant lies on the back with the legs elevated (see Figs. 2a and 3a). When the infant tends to hyperextend the neck, elevation of the pelvis must be increased. While lying on the back the infant is encouraged to reach towards the legs. A pronounced flexor pattern of the legs should be corrected to obtain extension of the knees in combination with hip flexion. Lateral weight shift and rolling is initiated from legs and pelvis while proper elongation of the neck must be obtained.

Handling

The infant is handled from arms and legs; when grasping around the forearms it is possible to apply traction downwards and outwards to counteract improper scapular elevation. The infant's open hands are placed behind and below the knees and the therapist supports both hands and legs with thumbs. To reinforce knee extension, the therapist places one finger on the thigh, above the knee joint (on the quadriceps muscles). During lateral rocking, attention is focused on maintaining good neck elongation.

Variation. The infant is only held around the arms. With the back of the fingers the therapist pushes the infant's elevated pelvis to one side initiating rolling and rotation within the body axis. Minimal support is given to obtain as much active participation as possible; rather than moving the infant back to midline, the therapist may want to wait for the baby to roll back (see Fig. 3b).

Righting Reactions of Head and Trunk in Sitting

Integration between flexion and extension in prone and in supine prepare trunk control in sitting. Before full integration between flexion and extension is developed, the baby sits in a ring sitting fashion: the legs are abducted and flexed at hips and knees, similar to the pattern assumed in supine during early hand to foot activities. By nine to ten months of age, the infant has sufficiently practiced differentiated leg movements in supine to be able to sit in a variety of postures with good sitting balance.

The hypotonic baby often sits with the legs in pronounced flexion/abduction and with an anterior pelvic tilt. With the trunk in front of the line of gravity, abdominal muscles are not activated for balancing and lateral righting is inhibited. In this case, head and trunk control must be prepared in supported sitting, prone, and supine as described above.

Some infants demonstrate lack of mobility which leads to insufficient hip flexion and causes the pelvis to be tilted too far back in sitting. In this case, elongation of the extensor muscles must be achieved in combination with

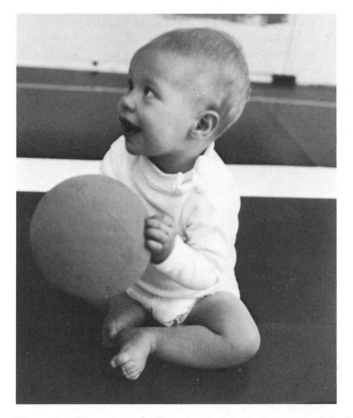

Figure 4a The extremely flexed and abducted posture of the legs interferes with the development of proper sitting balance (photograph by Carol Herwig).

facilitation of flexion against gravity as described in the activity for Integration Between Flexion and Extension in Supine.

The infant who has developed some degree of head and trunk control can be further challenged in righting and balancing while sitting.

Activities

In sitting, the baby is handled from the pelvis while the therapist displaces the center of gravity in every direction (Figs. 4a and b).

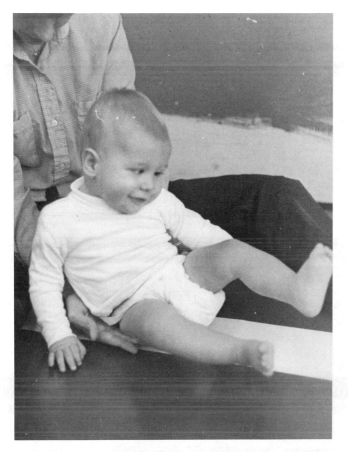

Figure 4b By handling the infant from the pelvis, the therapist can displace the center of gravity in every direction. The pelvis needs to be tilted back to achieve some flexion of the lumbar spine and subsequent activation of the abdominal muscles. To achieve axial rotation, the therapist should rotate the left side of this infant's pelvis backwards (photograph by Carol Herwig).

Handling

The therapist sits either behind or in front of the infant and places both
hands on the dorsal side of pelvis and hips while tilting the baby slightly back
into a posterior pelvic tilt so that the shoulders are behind the hips. The
weight is shifted laterally by elevating one hip. The non-weight-bearing side
of the pelvis should not be rotated forward because this results in hyperlordosis of the lumbar spine and reinforces predominant extensor patterns.
Trunk rotation can be elicited when the non-weight-bearing side of the pelvis
is slightly pulled back. When an additional stimulus for lateral trunk righting

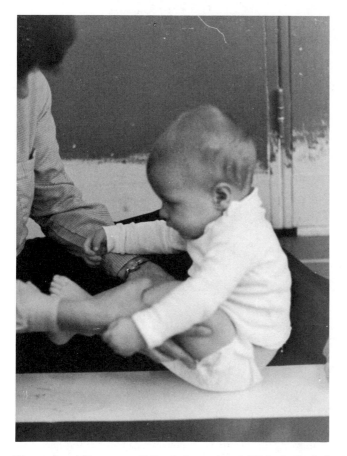

Figure 4c After some sitting balance is established, the infant can be handled from the legs (with a pillow behind the back, just in case!) (photograph
by Carol Herwig).

is necessary, the therapist applies a caudally directed pull from the lower rib-cage using the base or lateral side of the thumb. Initially, lateral oscillations should be minimal. When the infant is challenged beyond his or her limits, abnormal postural fixation may occur around the shoulders, arms and neck. With increased lateral weight shift the infant may place the hands down for propping.

When less assistance is required, the infant can be handled from knees or feet (Fig. 4c).

Variations. When proper trunk righting cannot be elicited using handling from pelvis and legs, the therapist facilitates axial extension and flexion with hands on the infant's trunk, i.e., on flexors and extensors.

The infant sits on the therapist's lap with face or back towards the thera-pist. Lateral weight shift is induced by the therapist elevating one leg and thus pushing the baby's weight to the downward side.

ROLLING AND CRAWLING IN PRONE

Mature patterns of rolling as well as normal patterns of belly crawling require a number of similar movement components. These include weight shifting through shoulder girdle, trunk, and pelvis, with active elongation on the weight-bearing side; lateral righting of head and trunk towards the non-weight-bearing side; and rotation within the body axis. All these movement components are reflected in the amphibian reaction where the weight-bearing side of the trunk elongates and the non-weight-bearing side shortens. At the same time, both limbs on the weight-bearing side extend and adduct while both on the other side flex. Excessive flexion or extension throughout the body inhibits the amphibian reaction, although many of these infants learn to roll or crawl but do so in an abnormal fashion.

Better function and quality of posture and movements can be prepared by facilitating the amphibian reaction as well as encouraging rotation within the body axis.

Amphibian Reaction

Appropriate elongation on the weight-bearing side is hampered by tightness in the shoulder girdle, especially between scapula and humerus. Full over-head flexion of the weight-bearing shoulder is inhibited by scapular protrac-tion and internal rotation of the shoulder.

Activities

The infant lies prone with both shoulders fully flexed and in slight external rotation. The arms rest on the supporting surface in neutral abduction or slight adduction. While the weight is shifted to one side, elongation of the weight-bearing side is initiated from shoulder and arm. Full flexion of the shoulder is rendered through a combination of shoulder, scapular, and spinal movement. Lack of mobility in the shoulder is often compensated for by excessive spinal extension. This must be corrected by aligning shoulder and pelvis. Proper weight shifting and lateral righting are further accentuated with reinforcement of the external rotation of the weight-bearing shoulder (Fig. 5a and b).

Resistance to full shoulder flexion is never counteracted by pulling on the arm. Sensory acceptance and preparation of tonus for this position are achieved when the infant is slightly rolled over the weight-bearing arm with the shoulder flexed to a degree which is comfortable. The therapist rotates the infant's shoulder back and accentuates weight bearing on arm and scapula with downward pressure.

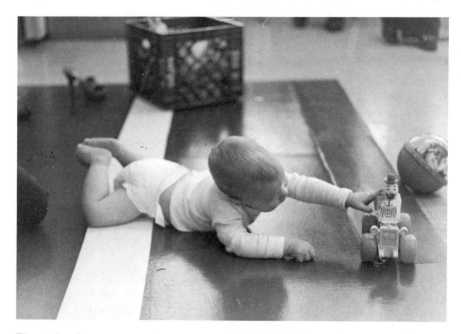

Figure 5a In contrast with the normal postural adjustments (amphibian reaction), head and trunk are flexed on the weight-bearing side—into gravity—while this infant reaches forward. Abduction of the limbs interferes with lateral weight shift.

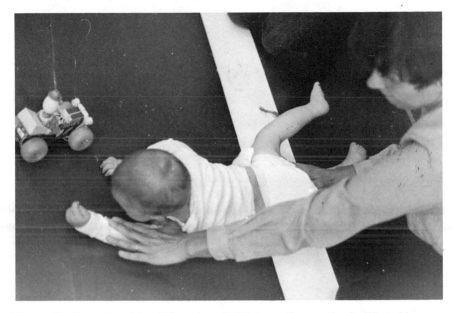

Figure 5b   Lateral weight shift and amphibian reaction can be facilitated by moving the weight-bearing arm into external rotation and adduction and the weight-bearing leg into internal rotation and adduction. The shoulder must be completely flexed (no space between axilla and support) (photograph by Carol Herwig).

Note: The hypotonic and hypermobile infant may lack proper response of the leg on the weight-bearing side. Instead of turning the leg towards internal rotation so that the foot points forward, the infant may maintain an extreme degree of external rotation. This must be corrected and proper postural adjustments need to be facilitated. Better support tonus on the weight-bearing leg is stimulated when the sensory feedback of weight bearing is accentuated by the therapist pushing the infant's leg and foot against the support.

Handling

In order to correct scapular protraction, the infant is handled from the shoulders. The sensory feedback of weight bearing on the lateral surface of scapula and humerus is accentuated with firm downward pressure. Lateral righting is facilitated by a slight pull in a caudal direction which is applied to the scapula and upper trunk of the non-weight-bearing side.

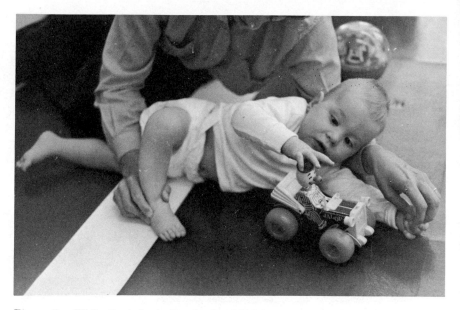

Figure 5c While the infant plays in the side lying position, the parent is shown how to facilitate proper upper extremity weight bearing while encouraging weight bearing on the contralateral foot. Note weight bearing on the lateral part of the foot due to external rotation of the hip (compare with Fig. 12b, Chapter 4) (photograph by Carol Herwig).

Variations. The amphibian reaction can also be facilitated from both limbs on the weight-bearing side or from the weight-bearing arm and contralateral leg (Fig. 5c).

When the above handling method does not produce sufficient trunk and hip flexion, the therapist changes hand placement to the weight-bearing shoulder and abdomen (Fig. 5d).

Carry-Over. The mother is instructed occasionally to place or carry the infant side lying (see Chap. 7) to reinforce the amphibian reaction.

Rotation Within Body Axis

Patterns of proper weight shift and lateral righting have been discussed for the supine, prone, and sitting positions (see activities for Lateral Head Righting, Integration Between Flexion and Extension in Prone, Righting of Head and Trunk in Sitting, and Amphibian Reaction). Lateral righting and rotation within body axis are also encouraged by placing the infant side lying.

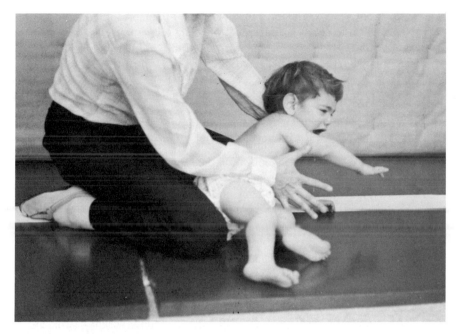

Figure 5d Rolling from prone to side lying, supine, or sitting is facilitated from the low rib cage and abdomen. To prevent shoulder and arm retraction on the non-weight-bearing side, the therapist extends fingers against the back of the infant's arm. This point of control is also used to shift the weight forward and to elicit rolling towards prone. At the same time the therapist retards the forward movement of the pelvis with the palm of the hand and thus encourages rotation within body axis (photograph by Carol Herwig).

There, patterns of extension and flexion are balanced allowing lateral flexion of the spine. When the infant moves towards prone, extension increases; when moving towards supine, flexion against gravity increases. Body righting on body leads to rotation and segmental rolling. When the fine interplay between flexion and extension is disturbed, postural alignment and balance during rolling are disturbed.

Activities

Side lying is a good position in which to start the facilitation of segmental rolling. Initially the excursions towards supine and prone are small. To prevent excessive extension of the spine, the shoulders lead when rolling towards prone, and the pelvis leads when rolling towards supine. The non-weight-bearing leg moves into flexion and adduction of the hip while rolling towards supine, and into extension and abduction while rolling towards prone. The weight-bearing arm is in alignment with the trunk: in full shoulder flexion and in some degree of external rotation.

Handling

Rotation of pelvis against shoulder girdle in prone to supine or side lying to sit is facilitated from the lower rib cage and abdomen.

Variation. For pronounced elongation between scapula and humerus, lateral flexion can be emphasized when the weight-bearing arm is raised off the support with the infant in side lying position.

UPPER EXTREMITY WEIGHT BEARING

Upper extremity functions, such as reaching, controlled arm movements in space and, finally, manipulative skills require postural stability of the shoulder girdle/trunk and dissociation of movements between head, shoulder girdle, and arms. These skills develop initially during activities of weight bearing. Some patterns of normal and abnormal upper extremity weight bearing are described in Chapter 4 ("Patterns of Upper Extremity Weight Bearing"). Efficient patterns of upper extremity weight bearing in prone are based on the ability to shift weight through trunk and pelvis. Without active hip extension, it is difficult to stabilize the pelvis for proper weight shifting.

Pelvic Control and Hip Extension in Prone

When head and chest are raised off the support active hip extension is apparent, first fleetingly and then more consistently by five to six months. Hip extension in space, such as lifting of the legs in prone, or in ventral suspension is a developmentally higher skill and develops later (six to eight months). The infant with delayed motor development keeps the hips in flexion and bears weight mostly on the chest while prone, and reaching activities are therefore hampered. In this case, weight bearing and weight shifting through the pelvis should be encouraged.

Activity

The infant is placed prone with shoulders fully flexed and externally rotated. The therapist is positioned in front of the infant, holding arms or hands, while encouraging the infant to lift head and chest off the support. The goal is to achieve a visible contraction of the glutei muscles. The infant should not be kept in a static posture. Small lateral weight shifts or rotation of head and trunk can be easily facilitated, especially when the infant lies on a large ball. Also, one arm may be brought down for propping while the infant is encouraged to reach with the other hand. Observe proper head righting with elongation of the neck.

Handling

The more distally the infant is held, and the less support is given, the more weight bearing occurs through the hips. When possible, the therapist supports the infant from the hands, holding him or her around the base of the thumb and the wrist to ensure wrist extension and abduction of the thumb in readiness for weight bearing on the hands. The palms of the hands are turned slightly toward each other to achieve external rotation at the shoulders. The infant should not use the distal support as a point of fixation, which may lead to a pull into flexion from the arms. This can be counteracted by giving only intermittent support. When more support is needed, the infant is held more proximally, i.e., by the shoulders and trunk. Elevation and protraction of shoulder and scapula can be inhibited and external rotation of the shoulder facilitated by encompassing shoulder girdle and arm.

Dissociation of Movements between Shoulder Girdle, Head, and Trunk

The infant with sensorimotor deficit often lacks the ability to dissociate movements between head, shoulder girdle, and trunk. Weight shift is often initiated from the head. The shoulder girdle cannot be stabilized and the scapula is thus pulled into protraction and elevation during arm and/or head movements. Appropriate righting of head and trunk is now inhibited.

Activity

The infant lies prone on forearms or hands on a mat, roll, or over the therapist's lap. Lateral weight shift through the trunk is facilitated by pushing in a diagonal direction, from one shoulder toward the opposite hip (Fig. 6a and b).

Handling

With both hands on the infant's chest and with extended fingers leaning against the frontal and upper part of the shoulder girdle, the therapist can correct scapular protraction and modify trunk responses.

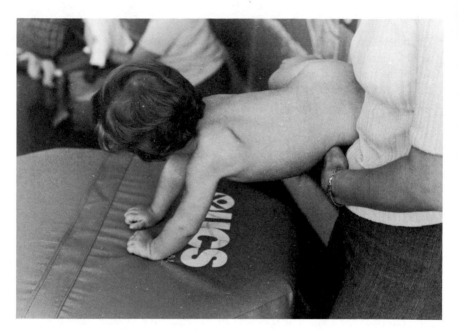

Figure 6a Poor shoulder girdle stability is indicated in the winging of the scapula. The posture of the left arm suggests some ATNR influence; the elbow is slightly flexed in combination with scapular protraction. The trunk sinks into gravity (lack of flexor component) (photograph by Carol Herwig).

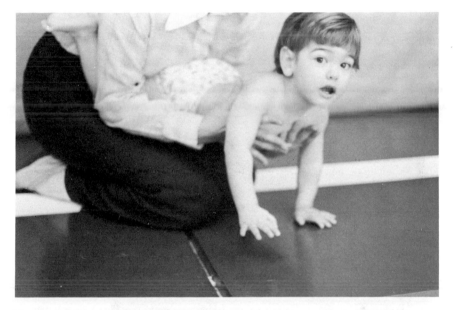

Figure 6b In prone on hands, better integration between flexion and extension can be facilitated by supporting the infant under the chest. With this point of control the therapist can also facilitate lateral trunk righting reactions when weight is shifted to one side. Support can be given at the lateral margin of the scapula (photograph by Carol Herwig).

**Upper Extremity Weight Bearing in
Reclined Sitting**

Activity

Proper patterns of weight bearing on elbows or hands and weight shifting can
also be carried out with the infant in reclined sitting. In this position, the
infant is encouraged to flex the head while extending the upper trunk. The

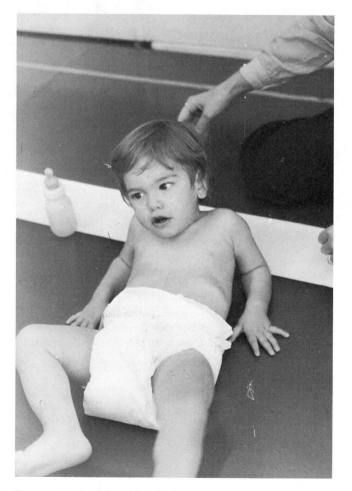

Figure 7a Poor shoulder girdle stability is especially obvious in supine on
arms and is combined with an inactive, "sagging" posture of the trunk. Note
the flaring of the ribs due to inactivity of the abdominal muscles (photograph
by Carol Herwig).

therapist should inhibit any tendency to scapular protraction and pronounced internal rotation of the shoulders. Upper extremity weight bearing should be carried out in various degrees of shoulder rotation. This helps to also prepare extension of the arms backwards where the shoulder is usually in a slight degree of internal rotation.

Handling

From shoulder girdle and upper trunk, the therapist can inhibit scapular protraction, accentuate weight bearing, and facilitate spinal extension and lateral weight shift (Fig. 7a, b, and c).

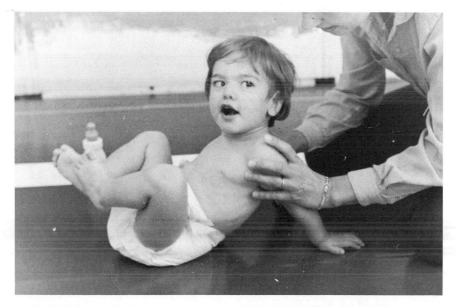

Figure 7b In order to achieve active control of shoulder girdle and trunk, the infant is handled from the shoulders (photograph by Carol Herwig).

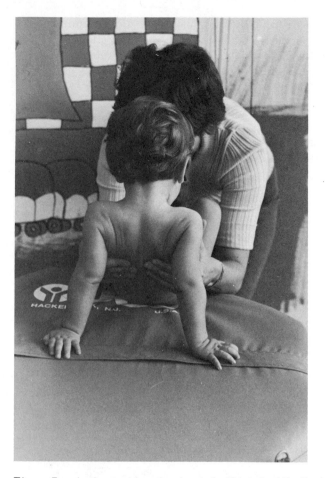

Figure 7c   Active trunk extension is facilitated while the infant is encouraged to right in the direction of flexion against gravity (photograph by Carol Herwig).

PROTECTIVE EXTENSION OF THE ARMS

Motor components required for protective extension are controlled extension against gravity and good stability of the shoulder girdle, combined with mobility and sufficient support tonus of the arms. Activities recommended in the section of upper extremity weight bearing prepare for protective extension of the arms. While the handicapped infant may prop on the hands, proper postural adjustments of head and trunk are lacking, especially in combination with lateral weight shifting. Shoulder girdle stability is also frequently impaired. The response may be delayed and support tonus of the arms is often insufficient.

Stability of the Shoulder Girdle

Moving the trunk around the weight-bearing arm is good preparation for the interplay between stability and mobility of shoulder girdle and arm.

Activity

With support under chest and abdomen, the infant is held in ventral suspension while leaning on both hands. The therapist induces lateral weight shift or axial rotation. During every phase of the activity, proper head righting must be facilitated and any tendency towards scapular protraction must be corrected. Shoulder girdle control is especially difficult when all the weight is resting on one hand as when turning from prone on hands to supine on hands (Figs. 6a, 8a to d).

Figure 8a With the support under the chest and abdomen, flexion, lateral flexion, or rotation of the trunk can be facilitated (photograph by Carol Herwig).

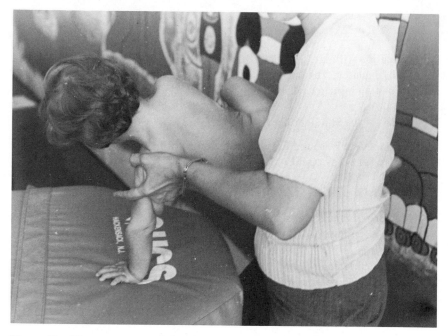

Figure 8b The grasp around the shoulder allows the therapist to correct posture of shoulder girdle and arm (photograph by Carol Herwig).

Figure 8c During the activity the therapist gradually reduces support and leaves more control to the infant (photograph by Carol Herwig).

Figure 8d Therapy must be dynamic and should consist of movement sequences, such as prone on hands to side propping to supine on hands and back. The difficulty of the task changes consistently and the therapist should be guided by the infant's response. For example, the further the body is shifted over the weight-bearing arm (forward, sideways), the greater the challenge (photograph by Carol Herwig).

Handling

The therapist gives support with one hand under chest and abdomen in order to monitor trunk responses, e.g., flexion, lateral flexion, elongation. The other hand is placed on the weight-bearing shoulder with the thumb on the ventral side of the shoulder to correct scapular protraction and elevation. The extended fingers lean against the infant's elbow to prevent collapsing of the arm, while the antihenar leans against the lateral margin of the scapula to inhibit pronounced abduction and winging of the scapula.

Variations. In prone as well as in side propping, the infant can be encouraged to reach in different directions including crossing of the midline.

When some shoulder girdle stability has been achieved, support from the upper trunk may be sufficient and can be substituted for direct handling from the shoulder girdle and arm.

Protective extension should be elicited in all positions and the therapist should vary speed and direction of displacement. Depending on the degree of postural control, the infant is handled from either proximal or distal points.

FOURPOINT-CRAWLING

Fourpoint-crawling is another big step in the infant's attempt to raise off the floor. It requires differentiation of movements and—with the pelvis off the floor—advanced skills of balancing. By the time the baby assumes fourpoint-kneeling (by about seven to eight months) equilibrium reactions have emerged in prone, supine, and possibly in sitting. Before fourpoint-crawling becomes an efficient means of locomotion, the infant has practiced balance by rocking in all directions while on hands and knees.

The infant with poor postural control keeps the center of gravity low while bearing most of his or her weight on the legs. This inhibits lateral weight shift and reciprocal leg movements.

To encourage proper crawling patterns, balance reactions are facilitated in fourpoint-kneeling (Fig. 9a,b,c).

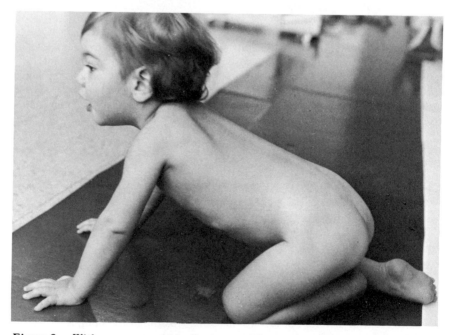

Figure 9a With pronounced hip flexion, weight bearing occurs predominantly on the legs, which inhibits lateral weight shift and frequently results in a pattern of "bunny hopping."

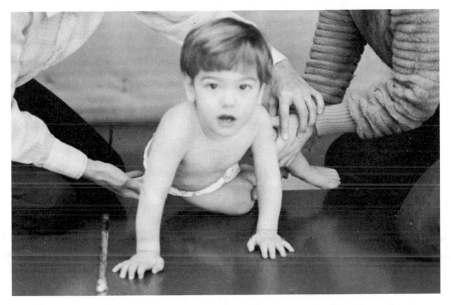

Figure 9b By correcting the leg posture, the parent can facilitate lateral weight shifting and axial rotation to prepare for reciprocal crawling (photograph by Carol Herwig).

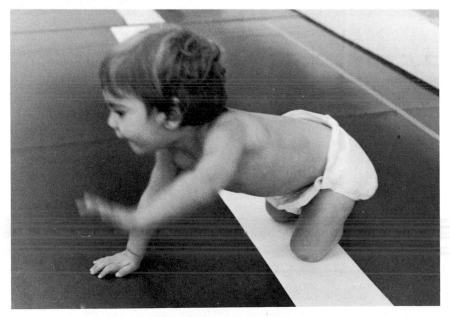

Figure 9c More appropriate postural tonus is indicated in improved postural alignment, balance, and distribution of weight bearing (compare with Fig. 9a) (photograph by Carol Herwig).

Pelvic Control and Balance Reactions in Fourpoint-Kneeling

Activity

The infant is placed on knees and hands with the legs in neutral abduction: knees under the body, and with knees and hips at about ninety degrees flexion. The therapist displaces the infant's center of gravity from the ventral side of trunk and pelvis or from the legs (Fig. 9b). Initially, the weight shift may be very small, until, later on, the infant can be moved between side sitting and quadruped position. Attention must be focused on adequate stability of the shoulder girdle and on proper rotation of pelvis and trunk. Any tendency to shoulder protraction must be discouraged. The weight-bearing arm should be vertical and, especially during rotation, the shoulder should not move forward in relation to the weight-bearing hand (see activities for Dissociation of Movements Between Shoulder Girdle, Head, and Trunk, and Stability of the Shoulder Girdle for handling techniques).

STANDING AND WALKING

Ambulation is a major concern to parents of infants with developmental delay. To help parents deal with this anxiety, the therapist should discuss with them the developmental stages infants must pass before they can take the first unassisted steps. It is often difficult for a lay person to accept that standing balance is not encouraged by placing the infant incessantly in an abnormal standing posture or being bounced on stiff legs. This may cause even further delay of balanced standing, especially when abnormal postural tonus is reinforced.

The fastest route to independent walking follows the course of normal development. Developmental stages of normal and abnormal patterns of standing and walking have been discussed in Chapter 4 ("Patterns of Standing, Supported, Unsupported"). In addition to the development of balance of head, trunk, and pelvis, the normal infant prepares the feet for weight bearing in various positions other than standing. When the infant finally pulls to standing, feet have acquired the necessary postural stability to carry the body weight while maintaining sufficient mobility to allow the gradual emergence of balance reactions.

The infant with poor postural tonus and abnormal motor patterns is frequently pulled into a standing position before the feet are properly prepared for the task. As a result, the weight distribution through the foot is abnormal which in turn affects the postural alignment of the body. Activities which encourage sensory awareness as well as balance reactions of the feet carried out in various positions other than standing help to diminish postural maladjustments in standing and walking. In addition, weight bearing in different degrees of hip and knee flexion (as for example, in the "bear position": standing on feet and hands), is especially helpful for the infant who tends to push into extreme extension or who locks the knees in hyperextension to achieve postural stability.

Foot-Eye Coordination

Normal infants (five- to six-months-old) engage in play activities with their feet while supine (legs in the air). They touch and handle feet, put toes into their mouths for investigation, and observe foot movements. The infant who lacks sufficient flexion against gravity is robbed of these opportunities. The developmentally delayed infant should be assisted in similar experiences and therapists should advise parents on how to incorporate "foot play" activities into their handling of the baby.

Activities

1. To facilitate lifting of the legs, the pelvis is raised while the infant lies on the parent's or therapist's lap or on a mat. To maintain the feet in the infant's visual field requires a combination of flexor and extensor patterns. Excessive hip flexion combined with abduction must be modified. The infant is encouraged to reach and touch feet and/or place toes in mouth. It is important to observe and inhibit any increased flexor tonus of arms while the infant holds on to the feet. In such a case, the baby is encouraged to touch the feet with open hands instead of grasping them.

2. Sensory awareness of the feet can also be reinforced when the infant is assisted in grasping soft objects, such as a small rubber or foam ball, using the feet. To enhance tactile and proprioceptive feedback, the therapist helps the infant to move the object between the feet. For correction of abnormal foot alignment see Handling as described in Weight Bearing on the Feet.

Weight Bearing on the Feet in Different Positions

Activities

Prone. Numerous prone positions lend themselves to weight bearing on dorsiflexed toes, e.g., prone propping, pivoting in prone, belly crawling, amphibian reaction (weight-bearing leg). In all these positions, the leg is extended, the ankle and the toes are dorsiflexed. The same posture is used, later on, for the push off phase in walking and represents a high level of postural differentiation. This posture contrasts sharply with the abnormal patterns of weight bearing on the toes where the ankle is in plantar flexion.

Handling

While the therapist pushes the infant's toes into dorsiflexion, he or she pulls the heel into elongation to achieve good dorsiflexion of the ankle. Pronounced forefoot pronation must be corrected. From the heel, some pressure is applied to reinforce weight bearing on the toes. It is absolutely essential that the foot be well-aligned when techniques of cocontraction are applied.

Side Lying Position. The normally developing infant often plays in side position on elbow or hand while using the upper, flexed leg for propping to give better postural stability (see Fig. 12b in Chapter 4). In this posture, the hip is in external rotation which allows weight bearing on the lateral border of the foot. This results in active lengthening of the lateral part of the foot while it encourages active lifting of the longitudinal arch of the foot.

The infant with sensorimotor deficits, if able to assume this position, uses internal rotation of the hip which leads to weight bearing on the medial border of the foot.

Handling

To encourage lengthening of the lateral and active shortening of the medial part of the foot, the therapist places the thumb against the medial surface of the calcaneus and the extended fingers against the lateral surface of the forefoot and the little toe. Any tendency towards internal rotation of the hip must be inhibited (see Fig. 5c).

Sitting. Partial weight bearing on the feet occurs in different sitting positions, especially in combination with weight shifting. When sitting on (note, not between!) the heels, the feet support almost the whole body weight (see Fig. 31 in Chapter 4). In this position the feet may be in plantarflexion or dorsiflexion of ankle and toes (see activity for Prone). Weight bearing on the feet can also be encouraged while the infant sits on a small stool or roll.

Handling

The therapist holds the infant's feet as described for activity for Side Lying Position. With the baby's feet well-aligned, the therapist bounces them repeatedly on the floor reinforcing proper weight bearing on the heel, lateral part of the forefoot, and all toes.

Balance Reactions of the Feet

Activity

In normal development, balance reactions of the feet are displayed in many different positions. Balance reactions of the feet deserve some attention in therapy, and should be encouraged during rolling, weight shifting in sitting, fourpoint-kneeling, knee-sitting, and so forth.

Handling

Different techniques of tapping can be applied either to the dorsiflexors of the ankle or to the plantar side of the toes to encourage dorsiflexion of the forefoot in combination with the appropriate balance reaction of the leg (abduction and flexion of the hip). Be careful not to elicit a positive support reaction by tapping on the ball of the foot.

Weight Bearing in Flexed Positions

Balance in standing and walking requires the ability to activate antigravity muscles while they are put into a state of dynamic elongation. This is difficult for a child with disturbed postural adjustments. Balance activities carried out in the "bear position," as on hands and feet, facilitate this skill and are, therefore, a good preparation for standing balance. The degree of flexion of hips and knees should be varied during the activity.

Activity

The therapist sits on the mat, with the infant, facing away, and on lap. Holding the infant around the knees, the therapist shifts the infant's weight forward and thus facilitates leaning on the hands. In this position, the baby is rocked in all directions, in straight planes as well as in diagonal directions, to encourage lateral righting and rotation within body axis (Fig. 10a and b).

Handling

The therapist puts one arm on each side of the infant's trunk and places the hands around the infant's knees to allow (a) the body weight to be shifted forward, which increases dorsiflexion of the ankles (one or two fingers are placed behind the knee); (b) inhibition of plantarflexion by providing downward pressure from the thigh (with the palm of the hand); (c) extension of the knees by pivoting the pelvis upwards and forwards (with the fingers placed underneath the thighs). Note that the knees should not be pushed into total extension because this leads to possible locking of the knees in hyperextension and to passive standing; and (d) inhibition of adduction of the legs (with thumbs on medial surface of thigh and knee).

Figure 10a Balance activities in the plantigrade position elicit activation of muscles while they are in a state of dynamic elongation (photograph by Carol Herwig).

Figure 10b Weight shifting is facilitated in all directions. For a description of different handling techniques, see Handling for Standing Balance (photograph by Carol Herwig).

Variation. When foot alignment needs correction, the therapist supports the feet with extended fingers while leaning the wrist or underarm on the infant's knees for control of the legs.

Standing Balance

Normally, an infant spends much time in supported standing, shifting the weight from foot to foot, twisting the body while letting go with one hand, or swinging one leg while trying to balance. Also, the infanct can bend over to pick up a toy or sit down. All these activities are preparations for independent walking. For the handicapped infant, standing experiences are often static. Body and legs stiffen and do not allow adequate balance responses. It is, therefore, important that the therapist provide such an infant with the experience of dynamic standing together with appropriate postural support and control.

Activity

The therapist sits on the mat, with the infant standing straddled over one leg. The therapist can modify support given to the infant by lowering or raising leg, grade the degree of hip and knee flexion when the infant sits down, or lift the infant in the air when the standing posture deteriorates. Undue hip adduction is also inhibited. In the standing position, the infant is gently pushed in all directions either through movements of the therapist's leg or through handling. During weight shifting it is important to facilitate proper rotation, as for example, trunk and pelvis rotate foreward on the weight-bearing side (Fig. 11a to d). In standing, the degree of hip rotation and abduction influences the foot posture. Hip adduction leads to weight bearing on the medial part of the foot. Pronounced external rotation also shifts the weight to the medial part of the foot. Internal rotation and flexion of the hip tend to shift the weight predominantly to the toes.

In treatment, the therapist facilitates a pattern of neutral or slight external rotation of the hips, unless the infant is in a step position where one leg assumes some degree of external rotation/abduction just before the push off phase.

Handling

The point of control asserted by the therapist depends on the infant's level of postural control. The more distal the point of handling, the more the baby has to balance. When foot alignment is poor and cannot be corrected bilaterally, the infant is brought to supported standing on one leg with the other knee leaning and bearing weight on the therapist's leg.

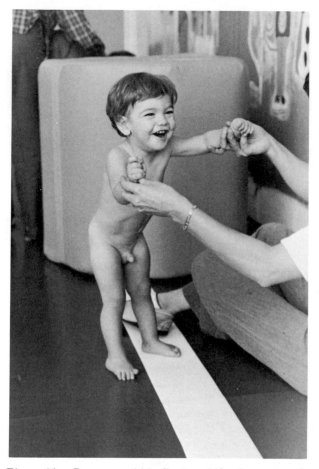

Figure 11a   Pronounced hip flexion shifts the center of gravity far back in relation to the base of support (feet) (photograph by Carol Herwig).

Variation.   When the infant is turned ninety degrees, the baby is in step position over the therapist's leg which permits weight shifting forwards and backwards (see Fig. 11d).

Facilitation of Walking

Correction of an abnormal gait pattern and facilitation of normal walking requires analysis and knowledge of the normal gait pattern. Walking requires a constant change in weight bearing. Before the initial step is taken, the weight must be shifted to one leg to free the other leg for the swing phase. In the mature gait pattern, the weight shift to one leg occurs with axial rotation: the

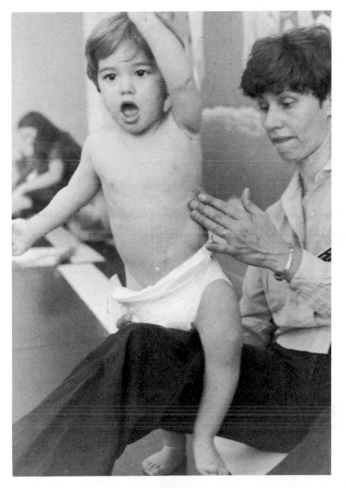

Figure 11b Hip extension is facilitated directly from the hip joint while the infant is also encouraged to rotate the non-weight-bearing side of trunk and pelvis backwards. When corrective support to the trunk is given on the weight-bearing side, the infant may lean into gravity rather than actively to right against gravity as happens when handled from the non-weight-bearing side (photograph by Carol Herwig).

weight-bearing side rotates forward, while the non-weight-bearing side rotates backwards. Next, the weight is transferred forwards. This occurs on the weight-bearing side, which means that the leg swings forward while the pelvis rotates backwards on this side until the heel strikes the ground. Now, a diagonal weight shift occurs, leading, again, to a forward rotation on the weight-

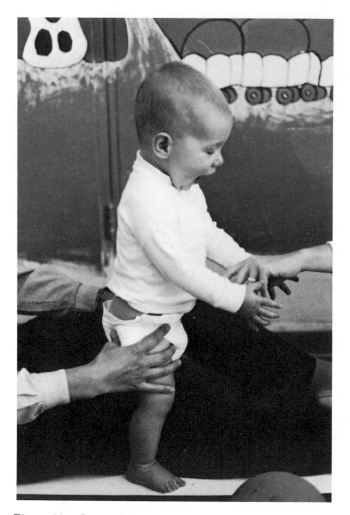

Figure 11c By straddling the infant over one leg during balance activities in standing, the therapist or parent can correct undue hip adduction, elicit lateral weight shift, or provide some standing support. Note well-integrated postural alignment throughout (photograph by Carol Herwig).

bearing side combined with the backwards rotation on the other side. The rotation of the shoulder girdle describes a larger amplitude and results, therefore, in some counterrotation between pelvis and shoulder girdle.

This degree of rotation within the body axis is absent during the infant's initial stages of unassisted walking. However, rotation within the body axis is practiced by the infant in supported standing even before venturing to take a first unassisted step. During facilitation of walking it seems acceptable to

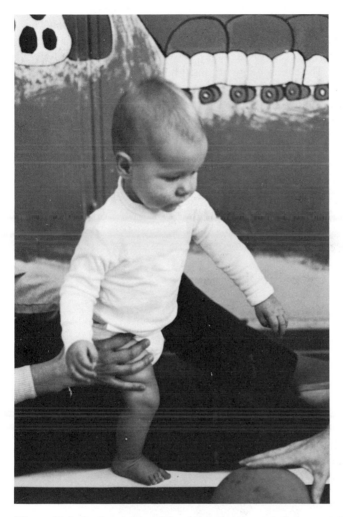

Figure 11d In the step position over the therapist's leg, axial rotation and external rotation of the hip are facilitated (photograph by Carol Herwig).

introduce a slight degree of rotation since the infant is given support. Careful grading of rotation is necessary to achieve proper postural alignment.

Handling

There are many ways of facilitating walking. The techniques used depend on the patient's skill in balance and postural alignment. It is not feasible here to describe more than one facilitation technique.

Substantial postural control can be achieved when the therapist walks behind the infant holding the shoulders and/or chest. For additional support
and control, the therapist can use the legs pressed against the infant's hips
and back (Fig. 12). The center of gravity must be aligned with the base of
support and the infant must never be allowed to lean or push back. While
shifting the weight, the therapist pushes down (diagonally) from the non-
weight-bearing shoulder and/or trunk for facilitation of lateral righting. At
the same time, this side is slightly rotated backwards while the weight-bearing

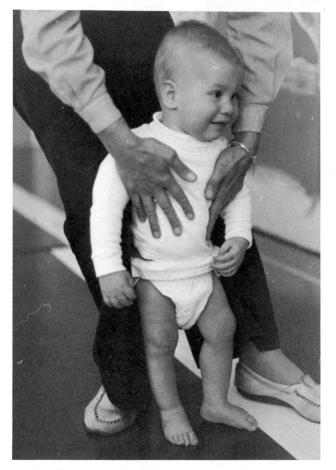

Figure 12 When substantial guidance and support are needed during walking,
the therapist can use the legs to bring the infant's hips forward while facilitating proper trunk righting and rotation as well as diagonal weight shifting with
hands on the infant's chest (photograph by Carol Herwig).

side is slightly rotated forwards. The therapist must facilitate the forward weight shift through the weight-bearing side. A common error is to push the pelvis forward on the side where the leg swings forward. This results in internal rotation of both hips and accentuates a frequently abnormal gait pattern. Support is, of course, gradually withdrawn in accordance with the infant's progress.

FACILITATION OF STANDING AND WALKING
AS PART OF THE OVERALL PROGRAM

Parents anxiously await the moment when their infant takes the first independent steps. This anxiety is, of course, even greater in parents of a handicapped infant and demands consideration by the therapist. However, there are dangers in pushing an infant toward independence. When the balance for standing and walking takes high priority in the treatment program, the quality of posture may be, to some extent, sacrificed.

Early phases of standing and walking are combined with a broad stance and symmetrical postures. The symmetrical and more primitive postures are, then, also applied in lower positions and the infant seems to regress in postural adjustments. It is, therefore, important not to work exclusively on standing and walking but to continue with some facilitation of mature postural reactions, such as axial rotation and differentiation of motor patterns in other positions that do not threaten the infant's balance.

SUMMARY

The goal of therapy is to provide the infant who demonstrates signs of CNS impairment with the experience of normal patterns of posture and movement. A major concern in all activities is the quality of motor patterns. Special emphasis is placed on proper postural alignment and well-integrated movement patterns of head and shoulder girdle which must be achieved to develop well-coordinated movements throughout the body (Fig. 13a to c).

The program design presented in this chapter focuses on some of the most important motor components and postural subskills of diverse functional activities. Handling techniques have been described in as much detail as possible in order to emphasize the importance of correct motor patterns.

It must be stressed that these activities are not applicable to each patient. The samples given must be adapted on an individual basis and the elicited responses must be critically assessed. Furthermore, therapy should offer the infant a vast variety of normal sensorimotor experiences far exceeding the examples given. The observation and analysis of normal motor behavior should serve as a guideline for the design of new activities.

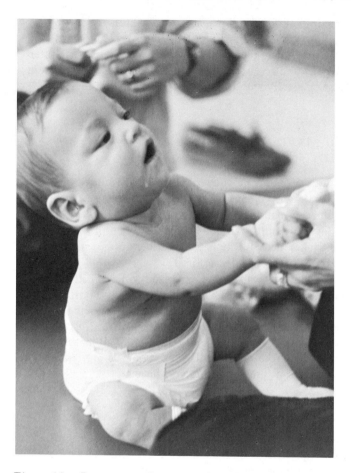

Figure 13a Poor postural control of head, shoulder girdle, and trunk severely restrict this eight-month-old infant in his interaction with the environment and further development in all areas.

Figure 13b Although his functional skills are not fully age-appropriate after twelve months of treatment, the displayed quality of postural tonus and alignment as well as the variability of his motor patterns indicate good integration of basic postural adjustments.

Figure 13c The foundation is laid for taking on the task of learning to master his environment.

Figure 13b

Figure 13c

The therapy approach to CNS dysfunction is still in a state of rapid growth and development. This poses exciting challenges to all professionals involved in the treatment of infants who display symptoms of sensorimotor impairment.

REFERENCES

1. Jackson, H. J.: Selected Writing of John Hughlings Jackson, Vol. 2. (James Taylor, Ed.). London, Staples Press, 1958.
2. Fisher, E.: Physiological basis of volitional movements, *Phys. Ther. Rev.* 38: 6, 1958.
3. Magnus, R.: Körperstellung. Berlin, Springer Verlag, 1924.
4. Schaltenbrand, G.: Normale Bewegungs– und Lagereaktionen bei Kindern. *Dtsch. Z. Nerv.* 87: 23, 1925.
5. Milani-Comparetti, A., Gidoni, E. A.: Pattern analysis of motor development and its disorders. Dev. Med. Child Neurol. 9: 625–630, 1967.
6. Bly, L.: The components of normal and abnormal movements during the first year of life. In *Development of Movement in Infancy* (Darlene Sekerak Slaton, Ed). Proceedings, University of North Carolina at Chapel Hill, Division of Physical Therapy, pp. 85–135, 1981.
7. Bobath, K., and Bobath, B.: The facilitation of normal postural reactions and movements in the treatment of cerebral palsy. *Physiotherapy* 50:246, 1964.
8. Quinton, M. B., and Köng, E.: Extensor 1-5, Baby Treatment. Film Kinderklinik, Inselspital, Bern. Maeder Film Limited, Basel, 1977.

BIBLIOGRAPHY

Bobath, B.: Treatment principles and planning in cerebral palsy. *Physiotherapy* 49:122, 1963.
Bobath, B.: The very early treatment of cerebral palsy. *Dev. Med. Child. Neurol.* 9:373-390, 1967.
Köng, E.: Very early treatment of cerebral palsy. *Dev. Med. Child Neurol.* 8: 198, 1966.
Köng, E.: Frühtherapy Zerebraler Bewegungsstörungen. *Med. Welt* 23: 446–448, 1972.
Köng, E.: Erfahrungen mit der Frühtherapy. *Paediatr. Fortbldg. Praxis* 40: 132-137, 1974.
Tauffkirchen, E.: Grundzüge der Physiotherapy bei Zerebralparese—nach Bobath. Paediatr. Praxis 16:539-549, 1975/76.

9
Assessment of the Management-Treatment Program

CONCEPT OF TREATMENT ASSESSMENT

Clinical appraisal of the results of surgical treatment in cerebral palsy patients is a well-established procedure [1]. Many of the evaluations have emphasized case reports and utilize follow-up studies. Up to the present, the approach has been similar although reviews of sizable samples are now more commonly employed [2] than individual case studies.

Effectiveness studies of nonsurgical and particularly multispecialty treatment approaches generally are a more recent development. The concept of formal therapy resulting in definitive change has been slow in developing. Rather, a variety of intuitive methods were applied almost more as a humanistic or charitable endeavor than a distinctive form of treatment. The approach to therapy detailed in Chapters 7 and 8 is the culmination and synthesis of advancement in theory and clinical practice to date. Its design for the individual patient today and its future applicability both rest on objective assessment procedures which can identify the influence of the treatment procedure itself in effecting developmental change. It is clear that many variables may play a part in the process of neurological growth and maturation.

Confirming the definitive role of a therapy program in affecting this process presents a major challenge to those whose clinical experience is devoted to this effort.

Two major issues are identified: (a) is the individual treatment program effective and appropriate for the given child? (b) is the treatment procedure substantiated by a body of data that includes long-term results? Evaluation of an individual treatment program must be based upon the following: (a) baseline developmental status of the child; (b) a total plan of care into which therapy is integrated; (c) management goals; and (d) treatment goals.

Individual treatment of the child should not be a separate and isolated procedure. It must realistically address the special needs identified in the evaluation; therapy should take its place among a variety of approaches which may include counseling and direction of parents, specialized design of physical features of the home as necessary, among many other possibilities. Most important, both short- and long-range goals developed must realistically relate to the needs of the child and the outlook for his or her future function. Goals for management and facilitation of child care must be considered equally with treatment objectives that may influence neurological change.

A procedure of regular assessment should therefore be part of the individual treatment regime. At periodic intervals it is essential to review changes in management problems, socialization, neurological status, and function ability in relation to objectives. Interviews with parents and other professionals can be used effectively to update documentation of management and social maturity. This could be further supplemented by psychological testing using such instruments as the Vineland Social Maturity Scale [3]. Clinical therapy evaluation of the infant should include assessment of tone, reflex behavior, developmental patterns of head and neck control, trunk stability, sitting, standing, use of extremities and walking, oral development, hand use, and perceptual ability. A specific format for reevaluation should be utilized to ensure uniformity and completness. An example of such a form in use is given in the Appendix.

On the basis of the clinical appraisal, judgment will be made either to continue or modify the treatment program, or its relationship to other influencing factors. Many intangibles must be considered including travel to the therapy site, the physical environment, and personality and relationship with the therapist. Any or all of these features or others may influence change and have an effect on outcome. The clinician must be in as objective a position as possible to decide whether a given program is adequately reaching the defined goals and when a change in emphasis or approach is indicated. The process of regular review needs to be included from the beginning in the procedure of working with the child.

The larger issue of long-term effectiveness of a given therapy procedure or approach and development of more effective methods continues to be an urgent professional need. As indicated in Chapter 3, several modalities are in current use. The general clinical impression from available studies using varying test instruments and designs is that early intervention is clearly related to neurological change in early follow-up [4-6]. However, data are totally lacking on the superiority of one method over another or of long-term effects. In more than thirty years of intensive therapy efforts up to 1966, only eleven major studies of effectiveness are noted by Wolf [7], and all have some serious defects in data or design. Possible relevant influence of family background and environment, supportive social and mental health services, improved neonatal care, and medical follow-up are among variables which may contribute significantly to a more favorable outlook for the affected child and are yet to be clearly delineated.

Perhaps we are now in a better position than ever before to identify and study the multiple factors using current computer technology. Moreover, the general climate of increased interest in and awareness of early identification and intervention has resulted in a proliferation of programs involving considerable numbers of children. The sizable populations participating in treatment programs offer the possibility of meaningful numbers for statistical analysis and detailed study, including large-scale collaborative efforts. Seriously lacking are effective instruments and procedures to gather the necessary data and study designs to ensure replicable research in a field committed to clinical service and long-term care.

ASSESSMENT PROCEDURES AND INSTRUMENTS

The first issue in studying the effects of therapy concerns use of evaluation procedures which will provide appropriate information about development and change. As our understanding of underlying neurological deficit and relevant variables has become more sophisticated so have the instruments and approaches to data gathering.

Narrative Reports and Case Histories

The simplest evaluation procedure is the narrative case report which generally reviews the patient's condition before and subsequent to a therapy program. Carlson was among the earliest workers to use this method of reporting [8]. The general format includes review of function in relation to therapy and the ascribing of change to the treatment procedure itself without necessarily considering the effect of growth, or comparing to a normal or even similarly handicapped patient. The case report continues to be used, often to substantiate a specific therapy modality [9-11].

Functional Inventories and Evaluations of
Activities of Daily Living

A variety of test instruments have been used to assess changes in functional ability, especially activities of daily living (ADL) in relation to therapy. Deaver was among the earliest to use an ADL test of function [12]. Brown expanded on Deaver's work and developed an Elementary Motor Skill Inventory for the young child, as well as a Daily Activity Inventory and Progress Record for older children [13]. These instruments were later modified for children with atypical movement [14], and for children with cerebral palsy in special classes [15].

Hoberman et al. found Brown's ADL Test inadequate for the preschool child and developed a Baby's Daily Activity Test. This was later modified into the Functional Development Motor Scale based on a comparison with the normal development scales of Gesell [16]. This was a prototype of several tests which attempt to assess function of the handicapped child in relation to a "normal" standard for age.

Ingram et al. developed a Cerebral Palsy Activity Record also primarily based on Gesell schedules. Assessment information enabled development of motor and social age quotients for children aged four weeks to five years [17]. Unfortunately, type and degree of neurological abnormality was not included for interpretation. Jones devised a developmental test and chart relating function to age using Gesell and other developmental components. This was especially scaled for cerebral palsy patients and provided for addition of serial data to monitor rate and type of change [18].

Anderson et al. also used a charting procedure to evaluate function and change in the areas of speech, hand use, balance, locomotion, and maturity [19]. Data enabled preparation of a profile for the child aged one month to four years. Footh and Logan later devised a Preschool Functional Activity Test specifically for the child with central nervous system deficit. It was an attempt to move away from simple Gesell norms and emphasized ability to adapt effectively, such as independently using a wheelchair [20].

Skill Tests

Crosland revised skill charts originally used by Phelps to analyze movement and range of motion [21]. Data were related to physical therapy procedures for tasks of lower extremities and to occupational therapy for activities of trunk and uppers. The tests were not graded by age and did not consider the quality of function.

Miller et al. also used a Motor Development Test of upper extremity activity [22]. This was related to an occupational therapy program.

Motor Ability Tests

Johnson applied the Gesell standards to a Motor Age test of extremity motor ability of children from four months to six years, who were compared with the normal [23,24]. The Bobaths later designed the Test Chart of Motor Ability [25], which was the first instrument to assess *quality* of movement and extent of abnormal postures in various positions. It was based on a normal developmental sequence and tests quality of function and developmental level rather than merely providing a physical measure of ability to function. Semans adapted the Bobath chart by arranging items in ascending order of complexity relative to central nervous system maturation with a grading system for each test item. Serial test profiles were used for assessment of change in motor ability [26].

Other motor development scoring systems have been in wide use. Zausmer and Tower developed a motor ability test as part of the American Academy for Cerebral Palsy's assessment instrument [27]. Scherzer et al. used a Motor Development Evaluation form grading presence and quality of motor patterns in prone, supine, sitting, quadruped, knee standing, standing, and walking. Presence and quality of primitive and postural reflexes were also included [28].

Development Profiles

Broad-scope assessment procedures involving various parameters of maturation have been utilized less frequently. Koven and Rowe prepared a five-point scale as a measure of degree of involvement. This included psychological and ambulatory status, ADL, and verbal ability [29]. No standardization was used.

Doman et al. have used several instruments to record related aspects of development. These include the Developmental Mobility Scale [30], the Doman-Moran Graphic Summary [31], and the Developmental Profile [32]. The latter records neurological integration based on developmental stages of motor, sensation, language, auditory, and tactile competency.

Pattern Analysis

Milani-Comparetti developed a chart to record patterns of movement (motoscopic observations) of trunk and extremities using notation similar to that used for choreography [33]. The record is to be used in comparison with notations of normal patterns.

A variety of visual methods have also been developed for recording and analyzing movement and, particularly, gait. These include light patterns [34], electromyography [35], and electronic or computer recordings [36], among others.

Clinical Assessments

By far the most commonly used procedure is general clinical assessment
without following a particular form, checklist, or formal test instrument. This
is similar to the individual case report but may have no specific outline or
form of reporting. It is a regular procedure of evaluation and reevaluation
practiced by therapists to update patient progress. It is also approached in almost as many diverse ways as there are therapists. Content is often not uniform even with the same therapist, in a given center, or even with the same
patient in subsequent reports. Therefore, it is often virtually impossible to
compare reports of an individual patient under treatment with a previous performance or to assess a relation with normal or similarly affected individuals.

There is a wide variety of approaches to recording information about patients. The focus may be narrow and involve motor skills alone or discrete
ADL functioning. It may broaden to include specific interrelated variables, or
generally consider the total development or function of a patient utilizing a
narrative case history. Many problems arise from the variety and types of assessments being used.

Lack of uniformity in reporting and use of several different test instruments within a therapy department of a treatment agency often prevents
meaningful analysis of change for a given patient. Comparing results with
patients from other agencies is further confounded by different types and
extent of data. As yet there seems to be little agreement on the type of reporting form and extent of information which should be included either in
the basic initial therapy work-up or in subsequent periodic reevaluations. This
may be a reflection of growth and maturation in this field. However, without
some generally agreed standards for data to be included in evaluations, the
goal of a rational approach to understanding objectively the effect of treatment and planning appropriate modification will remain illusory.

Many assessment instruments continue to be based upon the "normal" sequence of neuromotor development as set forth generally in the Gesell standards. A major inherent weakness is the simple transferral of data from such
standards to the developmentally impaired child [37]. Comparison with the
age-normal child, for example, does not provide an indication of rate and
quality of change. It may place the patient at continued disadvantage because
discrete areas of change often occur which have not yet become part of functional development. These would include more mature reflex behavior or improved range of motion which have not yet been incorporated into functional
activities.

Finally, objective reporting is often difficult to achieve. In the service-
oriented milieu, the therapist who has devoted much time, effort, and skill to
a patient cannot be faulted for being biased in favor of definite improvement
as a result of these efforts. Irrespective of the assessment procedure, form, or

test instrument used, if the observations are made by the treating therapist it is likely that such bias will affect the data to some extent. This may be further exaggerated by personality, and special interests of the therapist as well as program and budget considerations of the agency, among many possible factors.

SURVEY OF THERAPY STUDIES

An appropriate instrument to gauge the status of a child's development is a necessary and first condition in assessing individual progress and facilitating future treatment planning. That we are still far short of achieving this goal is amply demonstrated by the multitude of tests and procedures in current use, with their limitations.

Research on both effectiveness and value of the therapy approach itself is presently just emerging with some degree of scientific sophistication. A major limitation in the past has been inadequacy of available patient information, a direct result of previously discussed problems relating to test instruments and assessment procedures. In addition, studies of treatment have generally not had a specific design, but instead merely reported patient data from a particular form of therapy. Until relatively recently no consideration has been given to identification of variables other than treatment which could influence development. The influence of physiological growth alone has not been studied; control data have not been generated; long-term effects of treatment have not yet been considered. These are but a few of the concerns arising from lack of study design and presenting a major impediment to progress within this field. The types of study designs in use are reviewed below.

Narrative Case Reviews

Individual case histories and narrative case reports have already been considered as patient assessment instruments. Much of the "research" up to the present consists of such individual reports, often intending to substantiate one or another form of therapy. In some instances, these records have been brought together for numbers of patients to form a case review series. The individual clinical report serves as the data gathering method in a study design of case summaries. Information about outcome relates to motor development and functional ability.

Paine presented a classic case review follow-up study comparing "treated" with totally untreated patients known from 1930 to 1950 [38]. "Treatment" varied widely, was not consistent, and could not necessarily be well-documented, but was instituted in every instance at a relatively late age. Moreover, outcomes in neither treated nor untreated groups could be related to any of several possible associated variables such as age, intelligence, or degree of involvement. Under these circumstances it is not surprising that "treatment" seemed to make little difference for ambulation of the mild spastic hemiplegia patient on the one hand or for the severely involved athetoid patient on the other. Similarly, no specific effect of therapy was seen among those who had undergone orthopedic surgery.

Clinical case reviews of patients receiving specific treatment procedures include the early work of Kong [39]. Patients on Bobath treatment underwent repeat clinical evaluations after one to four years of therapy. Degree of involvement without indication of specific cerebral palsy diagnosis provided the basis for comparison. Satisfactory gait and minimal neurological signs were reported for this group. Woods did a similar clinical review of Bobath-treated patients and found a poorer prognosis for those with athetosis [40], but overall significant improvement in functional and neurological status.

Wright and Nicholson reviewed clinical findings on a group receiving a general physical therapy program [41]. Definite improved function is considered to be related to treatment itself. No analysis is given of other possible influencing variables.

Treatment Studies with Specific Assessment Instruments

Crosland reported the first study of treatment results with nonspecific therapy methods using *skill tests* [21]. No analysis was available of relevant variables. Both spastic and athetoid patients were reported to improve equally, and intelligence did not seem to be related to progress. Conflicting results were reported by Johnson using the *Motor Age Test* [24]. Here the data showed spastics responding better than athetoids; a higher IQ predicted better improvement; and many were thought to do as well without therapy. More responsive status for the spastic patient was again disputed by Ingram et al. using the *Cerebral Palsy Activity Record.* Patients were evaluated following intensive physical and occupational therapy.

Doman used a Mobility Scale to evaluate movement in children with mixed motor deficits receiving patterning treatment [30]. Encouraging results were noted. Again, no analysis of possible associated influencing factors is given, nor is there mention of possible effect of growth and maturation alone. Similar studies of this method using the expanded *Doman-Delacato Profile* of general function indicate improved rates of neurological growth [31,32]. However, analysis of patient background and environmental factors, among many other variables, is not available as in the initial study.

Adding to the inconsistent and often conflicting results with this group of studies is the work of Footh and Logan using the *PreSchool Functional Activities Test* [20]. They found no relationship to either previous or present physical therapy and no bearing of the IQ level on the effect of therapy.

Finally, Carlsen compared results of two occupational therapy procedures with young cerebral palsy children using perceptual and functional assessment evaluations [42]. Definite improved developmental levels were noted as a result of this early intervention.

Control Studies

Data from clinical evaluations, case reports, or the use of test instruments, leave undecided the question of placebo effect, or the role of growth alone, personality variables of the therapist, effect of the therapy visit itself, and many other possible confusing and conflicting factors which may color or influence any treatment regime. A research design which might resolve these concerns involves the use of controls. In this standard study design procedure two comparable populations are identified. One receives the treatment procedure while the other serves as a control (nontreated) group. Obviously, the closer the groups are matched, the more valid the comparison. Also, validity is enhanced if it is possible to mask the identity of treatment and control groups by physical separation, and appear to do similar things to both groups. This can be done by administering a "sham" procedure or similar device to the control group.

This classic approach has been the hallmark of scientific research into many areas of related medical fields. The need for such studies is readily apparent in the cerebral palsy treatment area. Research of this design is just now being developed.

Scherzer et al. used a double-blind research design to study the effect of physical therapy on cerebral palsy children under eighteen months of age [28]. The treatment group received a combination of several presently accepted modalities of neurodevelopmental physical therapy; the control group utilized traditional passive range of motion exercises only. Assignment to groups was by random selection. Group matching was not attempted due to small sample size. Evaluating therapists and physician were unaware of group assignments. A motor assessment instrument previously described was used to determine changes in motor status. Social change was determined through the Vineland Social Maturity Scale. Effect on home management was evaluated through pre- and post-test questionnaires completed by patients' families. In each of these areas the treatment group showed significant improvement.

Hochleitner then studied comparable groups of cerebral palsy patients with and without Bobath therapy [43]. No specific test instruments are described. Direct matching of the two groups was also not attempted. Cerebral palsy diagnoses varied as did severity and associated disabilities. Results of long-term follow-up show significant reduction in disability among the treatment group while controls continued with severe deficit. The initial severity of both groups is not given and could be a factor in later results if those who were initially more involved fell into the nontreated category. Nevertheless, those subjected to therapy clearly had significantly less residual disability when reevaluated.

The control study design approach clearly offers many advantages in singling out the effect of the therapy procedure as the variable most directly related to change. However, much depends on the validity of the assessment instruments, comparability of the groups being compared, elimination of observor bias and other possible influencing factors.

Other Studies

Rembolt has developed an extensive compendium of research in recent years in the categories described, with the exception of control studies [44]. An explosion of treatment investigation parallels the current trend toward early intervention in all types of developmental disabilities, often in young infants on whom a definitive neurological label cannot be placed [45]. More sophisticated control designs are replacing case studies and narrative reviews; [46] and computerization of data is enabling greater precision of multivariate analysis [47].

Status of Cerebral Palsy Research

The multihandicapping nature of cerebral palsy accentuates the problems of identifying both discrete and interrelated areas of development responding to treatment. Change occurs slowly and simultaneously with parallel growth and maturation. Identification and objective measurement of specific aspects of the child's functioning remain elusive but are necessary first steps in any meaningful study. The data are "soft" because quantitative measurement is generally not possible. One must resort to semiquantitative scales and descriptive profiles derived from many units of information.

Current evidence on the effect of early treatment in cerebral palsy is weak but thought-provoking, with clear trends confirming its validity. The evidence remains "soft." Sampling size has been insufficient in reports from many different geographical and environmental backgrounds. Comparability has not been possible due to lack of standardization in treatment procedures, types of evaluations, or reporting. Bias in sampling and evaluation remains the rule. Too little attention has been given to objective recording in evaluations. Use of varied methods of data gathering such as questionnaires, interviews, and physiologic measurements has been frequently neglected as a variable. Only recently has study design itself been emphasized. Fortunately, considerable impetus for improvement is now coming from the work in developmental psychology and early intervention studies of the developmentally delayed child.

A word must be said about parental expectation and evaluation. However the professionals may view the effect of a given therapy in general or in a particular child, at any point the parent will view developmental change in relation to preset goals and expectations of the therapy procedure. The value of treatment is still more extolled than proven and often turns on the convictions and personality of the therapist. Both may vary and change with individuals and as yet the parent must pursue through faith rather than hard data. This is the challenge for those whose clinical experience has confirmed the value of early treatment approach described in Chapters 4 to 8.

DEVELOPING EFFECTIVE STUDY DESIGNS

Review of some current studies has shown encouraging trends in effecting developmental changes through early intervention therapy. Validity of the data remains in question, however, because of weaknesses in the quality and objectivity of information, the inability as yet of totally excluding interference from other possible factors which may cause change, and designs which do not fully enable comparison with those left untreated. That these conditions continue in spite of highly sophisticated research efforts in today's behavioral sciences and related "soft data" fields is a reflection of the special circumstance of this service-oriented field. The problem of demonstrating irrefutable evidence that early therapy makes a significant difference remains after years of treatment efforts. This base must first be fully established. Having done so the next and persistent challenge will be to determine which types of therapy and special conditions are most appropriate for a particular child with specific deficits; that is, the search for a discrete prescriptive approach to treatment based on known effect and long-term follow-up. These goals may, in fact, be attainable if we can understand better the special conditions, problems, and obstacles which are likely to affect any research effort in this field.

Research Obstacles

THERAPISTS IN THE RESEARCH MILIEU
Therapy is committed to servicing and treating those in need. It is an action-oriented profession. As in any clinical setting, the *personality of the therapist* may have a major bearing on the response of the patient, *no matter which procedure is being followed.* From the very beginning, therefore, an element of influence may be introduced whose effect could be crucial. This is a variable which will have to be anticipated and "controlled" or at least recognized in any study of treatment results.

Because therapists are caring individuals and closely associated with a particular type or school of therapy, they are convinced their treatment will work and will be beneficial to patients even before starting. This is especially and increasingly true today as many centers are exclusively providing a particular form of treatment such as neurodevelopmental therapy (NDT).

The therapy program is often viewed by the therapist as a unique and specific treatment in itself, comparable to a dose of medication. Often it is not placed in the perspective of an approach requiring practice and carry-over at home or a direction for behavioral stimulation, which is generally regarded as its basis of operation. To withhold treatment from some or to modify conditions to enable study is for many therapists at best a rejection of their perceived role and at worst a deception of the patient or family. No wonder the therapist often objects to studies in which there is selection and control of patients or where the conditions require some alteration from the accustomed treatment regime.

Finally, the therapist often develops a unique rapport with the family and is the major avenue of communication for anything which influences the child. A perceived alteration in treatment required for study purposes or a negative response by the therapist to a study procedure, could be quickly recognized by the parent and affect much-needed cooperation.

The focal role of the therapist as an influential committed individual must be fully delineated and respected. When this issue is fully understood it will be possible to utilize the inherent strengths of therapy staff to help design and participate in more objective approaches to understanding the effects of treatment.

CONTROLLING ENVIRONMENTAL AND OTHER INFLUENCES

The therapist is one of several major variables which may affect developmental change. Home conditions, interest, adjustment and response of family members, particularly providing stimulation, and in expectations, are also among the most potentially relevant. An accurate picture of these factors is essential so that their possible or potential effect on the child's development can be assessed in relation to the treatment procedure and results.

SAMPLING

A major problem is that frequently only small numbers of children are under treatment in a given center or program. This may be a reflection of a relatively small infant population in some areas or limited referrals of very young children with suspected early developmental deficits. The latter continues to be a major problem stemming from limited awareness of early identification by practitioners and/or lack of conviction of the value of early intervention. The sample size will therefore often not enable matching, comparing, control designs, or other means of statistical design. It is also often not possible to deal with narrow ranges of homogeneous age, diagnosis, or degree of disability ranges, and instead more heterogeneous groupings must be used. This reduces the ability to deal specifically with unique groupings and the resulting data often becomes far too general.

A possible solution to this type of problem is the organization of large-scale collaborative studies. Comparable groups are identified in multiple centers, each receiving identical interventions under conditions which are comparably controlled. By this means, sufficiently large numbers of subjects under investigation enable use of sophisticated statistical techniques. This procedure is already well-established in several areas of medical care including treatment of renal disease [48], leukemia [49], and in the previous collaborative maternal and infant study of cerebral palsy etiology [50].

SELECTING AND USING TESTING INSTRUMENTS

Much has already been said about the problems in collecting data and information relating to developmental change. Uniformity is the greatest need in developing initial and follow-up evaluations so that records are complete and comparable. The assessment instrument to be used is often selected on the basis of "normal" developmental standards and frequently does not allow an adequate understanding of rate of change for a given individual irrespective of chronological expectations. Also assessments may depend heavily on only the clinical judgment of the evaluating professional without specific objective measurement guidelines.

RECORDING AND INTERPRETING DATA

Observer bias is the single most difficult research obstacle with which to deal. Even after many hours dedicated to treating patients therapists can be convinced that their prescribed treatment is most effective with no need for an alternative approach. A possible solution is to use another therapist to perform reevaluations, and record and interpret the data regarding developmental change. This could have many obvious advantages, not the least of which is to encourage more objective reporting.

USE OF CONTROLS

Many of the studies reported have an inherent design of comparing the patient with his or her previous level of development and function. This is a well-established procedure in which the individual is used as his or her own control [51]. While this method gives the appearance of an effective objective procedure, it has some definite weaknesses. Firstly, since the initial or previous evaluation numerous factors other than the treatment procedure itself could be operative in effecting change. These might include changes in environmental conditions, such as parental interest or support, physical developmental acceleration, or the addition of other environmental stimulation not previously available. Clearly, it must be specifically ascertained that, during the periods being compared, changed conditions or other possible influencing variables can be discounted.

Actual matched control studies of early intervention therapy are just now beginning to emerge, as previously discussed. The limitations relate to frequent small sample size which prevents effective matching, resistance by therapists and other staff to withholding any treatment from young children for the sake of research, and the ever-present difficulties of selection of appropriate assessment instruments and reducing bias in reporting. Each of these can be dealt with if the involved professional is aware of the implications of his or her role and can grasp the advantages of achieving reputable research findings to substantiate the place of therapy in affecting development of infants with neurological deficit.

Planning for Effective Patient Assessments

The following is a suggested guide to the clinical approach to patient assessments. The need for reasonable completeness, uniformity, consistency, and objectivity pervades all facets of the evaluation of patients. The extent to which these guidelines are followed will determine potential for accurate long-term follow of individual patients as well as ultimate comparability among groups of children being treated at numerous centers.

INITIAL EVALUATION

1. Schedule adequate time for a full evaluation schedule to meet the specific goals of the therapy program.

2. Provide an appropriate, reasonably quiet place where interruption will be minimized.

3. Predetermine specific areas of development to be assessed: consider confining evaluation to one or more of the following:
   a. Motor development
   b. Functional ability—ADL
   c. Social maturation—management level
   d. Oral development/speech.

4. Prepare assessment form in outline, if possible, with check-off design.

5. Summarize findings, short- and long-range therapy goals, and plan of treatment.

6. Plan in advance for schedule of reevaluation assessments

7. Review plans with other therapies for gaps and overlap in treatment. The combined effect is to prepare for each child an Individual Development Plan (IDP)

REEVALUATIONS

1. Set aside regularly scheduled periods in quiet conditions for reevaluations.

2. Develop a suitable reevaluation form in check-off style, if possible, for each developmental area being considered.

3. Summarize findings: prepare new short- and long-range goals, revising previous plans as appropriate.

4. Maintain regular schedule of reevaluations using prepared forms. Suggested intervals would be more frequent with very young children (about every three months), and less often as the child grows. Examinations should be at least twice annually.

5. Continue regular joint reevaluations with entire therapy team for full review and planning.

The goal is for all therapists to develop an appreciation of the objective and thorough evaluation process as a major integral professional responsibility. Without question this is on a par with actual physical contact and treatment of the patient.

Guidelines for Therapy Research

Adequate assessments, instruments, and procedures are a first requirement in developing objective information on the child's level of development and function. Only after these are developed can study be initiated on the effects of a particular therapy modality. While practitioners must be aware of the obstacles and difficulties inherent in research in this area, the following guidelines are offered for those who have an interest in planning research or better interpreting and understanding research reports:

1. Gain the interest, confidence and acceptance of staff through frank discussion of the need and purposes of research studies.

2. Begin any study with an objective outlook toward the benefit of a treatment procedure.

3. Develop a design which will avoid or eliminate possible interfering environmental influences and other spurious variables.

4. Consider the use of control designs with matching of samples if possible.

5. Use a large enough sample to develop the data properly. Consider possible data sharing and collaboration with other comparable centers. Use objective random or other statistically valid sampling techniques.

6. Select assessment instructions for objectivity, completeness, and relevance to research goals.

7. Utilize objective therapist evaluations by nontreating therapists where possible.

8. Obtain results of parent, teacher, and other relevant professionals' interviews and questionnaires both prior to and during therapy to develop information about expectations and outcomes.

9. Be consistent in following out the research design with proper sampling assessments and objective recording of data until required sample number is complete.

While no single set of guidelines will assure quality of research, it is clear that a well-prepared and executed design is the best hope for a meaningful study. This is clearly a major need in the therapy field and could do much to strengthen standards for treatment and professional growth. A solid research foundation is the necessary ingredient to firmly establish the relevance of both early evaluation and infant intervention programs.

APPENDIX Reevaluation

Name: Chart No.:   Birth Date: Date: Therapist:

Date of Last Report:

I.   Summary of Last Report:

II.   Program Goals of Last Report:

III.   Changes of Behavior as Compared with Last Report

     1.   Functional Abilities:

     2.   Motor Patterns

         Normal Postural Adaptations (Righting reactions, head control, postural symmetry and midline control, shoulder girdle stability, trunk control and proximal stability, protective extension of the arms, equilibrium reactions, manipulation and eye-hand-foot coordination, differentiation and variability of movements):

         Abnormal Postural Responses (exaggerated tonic reflexes, predominant hyperextension of head and neck, predominant scapular protraction/retraction, total and ungraded extensor patterns, pronounced/compensatory flexion, pronounced anterior/posterior pelvic tilt, stereotyped behavior, paucity/excess of movements):

Postural Tonus (normal, hypotonic, hypertonic, rigid, fluctuating, associated reactions)
At rest:
Changes in response to stimulation, handling, movement:

3. Overall Quality of Motor Behavior (variability, grading, sequencing):

4. Predominant Motor Patterns:

5. Restricted Mobility, (Risk for) Contractures, Deformities:

6. Reaction to Sensory Stimulation (kinesthetic, tactile, auditory, visual):

IV. Additional Comments:

V. Summary:

VI. Program Goals:

VII. Recommended Procedures:

REFERENCES

1. Green, W., and McDermott, L.: Operative treatment of cerebral palsy of the spastic type. *JAMA* 118: 434, 1942.
2. Couch, W., De Rosa, G., and Throop, F.: Thigh adductor transfer for spastic cerebral palsy. *Dev. Med. Child Neurol.* 19:343, 1977.
3. Louick, D., and Boland, T.: Psychologic tests: A guide for pediatricians. *Pediatr. Ann.* 7:86, 1978.
4. Barrera, M., et al.: Early Intervention with biologically handicapped infants and young children: A preliminary study with each child as his own control. In Tjossem, T. (ed): Intervention Strategies for High Risk Infants and Young Children. Baltimore, University Park Press, 1976, pp 609-627.
5. Hayden, A., and Haring, N.: Early intervention for high risk infants and young children: Programs for Down's syndrome children. In Tjossem, T. (ed): Intervention Strategies for High Risk Infants and Young Children. Baltimore, University Park Press, 1976, pp. 573-607.
6. Aronson, M., and Fallstrom, K.: Immediate and long-term effects of developmental training in children with Down's syndrome. *Dev. Med. Child Neurol.* 19:489, 1977.
7. Wolf, J.: The Results of Treatment in Cerebral Palsy. Springfield, Chas. C Thomas, 1969.
8. Carlson, E.: Motor re-education in birth injuries—a case report. *Yale J. Biol. Med.* 3:49, 1940-1931.
9. Wainer, G.: Psychotherapy in a girl of 18 years with severe cerebral palsy. *Dev. Med. Child Neurol.* 7:175, 1965.
10. Spira, R.: Management of spasticity in cerebral palsied children by peripheral nerve block with phenol. *Dev. Med. Child Neurol.* 13:164, 1971.
11. Skrotzky, K., Gallenstein, J., and Osternig, L.: Effects of electromyographic feedback training on motor control in spastic cerebral palsy. *Phys. Ther.* 58:547, 1978.
12. Deaver, G., and Brown, M.: Physical Demands of Daily Life. Studies in Rehabilitation No. 1. New York. Institute for Crippled and Disabled, 1945.
13. Brown, M.: Daily activity testing and teaching. *Phys. Ther. Rev.* 27: 249, 1947.
14. Brown, M.: Daily activity inventory and progress record for those with atypical movement. *Am. J. Occup. Ther.* 4:195, 1950.
15. Brown, M.: Daily activity inventories of cerebral palsied children in experimental classes. *Phys. Ther. Rev.* 20:415, 1950.

16. Hoberman, M., Cicenia, E., and Stephenson, C.: A useful measurement tool in the physical rehabilitation program of pre-school orthopedically handicapped children. *Arch. Phys. Med.* 32:457, 1951.

17. Ingram, A., Withers, E., and Spetz, E.: Role of intensive physical and occupational therapy in the treatment of cerebral palsy: Testing and results. *Arch. Phys. Med.* 40:429, 1959.

18. Jones, M.: Appraisal of Progress in the Cerebral Palsied Child. Los Angeles, United Cerebral Plasy of Los Angeles County, 1952.

19. Anderson, R., Bargowski, E., and Blodgett, W.: A Code Method for Evaluating Function in Cerebral Palsy. Detroit Orthopedic Clinic, 1961.

20. Footh, V., and Logan, K.: Measuring the effectiveness of physical therapy in the treatment of cerebral palsy. *J. Am. Phys. Ther. Assoc.* 43:867, 1967.

21. Crosland, J.: The assessment of results in the conservative treatment of cerebral palsy. *Arch. Dis. Child.* 26:92, 1951.

22. Miller, A., Stewart, M., Murphy, M., and Jantzin, A.: An evaluation method for cerebral palsy. *Am. J. Occup. Ther.* 9:105, 1955.

23. Johnson, M., Zuck, F., and Wingate, K.: The Motor Age Test: measurement of motor handicaps in children with neuromuscular disorders such as cerebral palsy. *J. Bone Joint Surg.* [Am] 33:698, 1951.

24. Johnson, M.: The use of the Motor Age Test in the evaluation of cerebral palsy patients. Instruct. Lect. Am. Acad. Orthop. Surg. 9:108, 1952.

25. Bobath, K., and Bobath, B.: An assessment of the motor handicap of children with cerebral palsy and their response to treatment. *Am. J. Occup. Ther.* 2:19, 1958.

26. Semans, S.: A cerebral palsy assessment chart. *J. Amer. Phys. Assoc.* 45:463, 1965.

27. Zausmer, E., and Tower, G.: A quotient for the evaluation of motor development. *J. Am. Phys. Ther. Assoc.* 46:725, 1966.

28. Scherzer, A., Mike, V., and Ilson, J.: Physical therapy as a determinant of change in the cerebral palsied infant. *Pediatrics* 58:47, 1976.

29. Koven, L., and Rowe, R.: A general capacities scale for children with neuromotor handicaps. *Am. J. Occup. Ther.* 13:166, 1959.

30. Doman, G., Delacato, C., and Doman, R.: The Doman-Delacato Developmental Mobility Scale. Philadelphia, The Rehabilitation Center, 1960.

31. Doman, G., Delacato, C., and Doman, R.: The Doman-Delacato Developmental Profile. Philadelphia, The Rehabilitation Center, 1962.

32. Doman, G., and Moran, P.: The Doman-Moran Graphic Summary. Philadelphia, The Institutes for the Achievement of Human Potential, 1963.

33. Milani-Comparetti, A., and Gidoni, E.: Pattern analysis of motor development and its disorders. *Dev. Med. Child Neurol.* 9:625, 1967.

34. Aptekar, R., Ford, F., and Bleck, E.: Light patterns as a means of assessing and recording gait. II results in children with cerebral palsy. *Dev. Med. Child Neurol.* 18:37, 1976.
35. Csongradi, J., Bleck, E., and Ford, F.: Gait electromyography in normal and spastic children, with special reference to quadriceps femoris and hamstring muscles. *Dev. Med. Child Neurol.* 21:738, 1979.
36. Close, J.: Motor Function in the Lower Extremity: Analyses by Electronic Instrumentation. Springfield, Chas. C Thomas, 1964.
37. Semans, S.: Specific tests and evaluation tools for the child with central nervous system deficit. *J. Am. Phys. Ther. Assoc.* 45:457, 1965.
38. Paine, R., On the treatment of cerebral palsy: The outcome of 177 patients, 74 totally untreated. *Pediatrics* 29:605, 1962.
39. Kong, E.: Very early treatment of cerebral palsy. *Dev. Med. Child Neurol.* 9:198, 1966.
40. Woods, G.: The outcome of physical treatment in cerebral palsy. *Cerebral Palsy Rev.* 25:3, 1964.
41. Wright, T., and Nicholson, J.: Physiotherapy for the spastic child—an evaluation. *Dev. Med. Child Neurol.* 15:146, 1973.
42. Carlsen, P.: Comparison of two occupational therapy approaches for treating the young cerebral palsied child. *Am. J. Occup. Ther.* 29:267, 1975.
43. Hochleitner, M.: Vergleichende Untersuchung von Kindern mit zerebraler Bewegungsstörung, mit und ohne neuro-physiologischer Fruhtherapie. *Oestr. Aerzt.* 32:1108, 1977.
44. Rembolt, R., and Roth, B (eds)· Cerebral Palsy and Related Developmental Disabilities—Prevention and Early Care. An annotated Bibliography, Vols. I–III. Columbus, Ohio State University Press, 1975.
45. Tjossem, T. (ed): Intervention Strategies for the High Risk Infant. Baltimore, University Park Press, 1976.
46. Leib, S., Benfiedl, G., and Guidubaidi, J., Effects of early intervention and stimulation of the pre-term infant. *Pediatrics* 66:83, 1980.
47. Zar, J.: Biostatistical Analysis. Englewood Cliffs, N.J., Prentice-Hall, 1974, p. 190.
48. Spitzer, A et al: Prospective controlled trial of cyclophosphamide therapy in children with nephrotic syndrome. A report for the Information Study of Kidney Disease in Children. *Lancet* 2:423, 1974.
49. Miller, D.: Prognostic factors in childhood acute lymphoblastic leukemia. *J. Pediatr.* 87:672, 1974.
50. Nelson, K., and Ellenberg, J.: Neonatal signs as predictors of cerebral palsy. *Pediatrics* 64:225, 1979.
51. Martin, J., and Epstein, L.: Evaluating treatment effectiveness in cerebral palsy: single-subject designs. *Phys. Ther.* 56:285, 1976.

Author Index

Numbers in brackets are reference numbers and indicate that an author's work is referred to although his name is not cited in the text. Italicized numbers give the page on which the complete reference is listed.

Accardo, P., 6[14], *16, 143*
Adran, G. M., 58[9], *69, 202*
Amatruda, C. S., 21[1], 48[1], *51, 122, 143*
Anderson, R., 260[19], *276*
André-Thomas, *122, 142*
Andrews, B., 13[64], 14[64], *19*
Aptekar, R., 261[34], *277*
Aronson, M., 259[6], *275*
Ashby, S., 13[68], *19*
Ashworth, M., 11[49], *18*
Autgaerden, S., *122, 142*

Bandera, E., 11[38], *17*
Bandura, A., 67[42], *71*
Bargowski, E., 260[19], *276*
Barnett, H., 13[62], *18*
Barrera, M., 259[4], *275*
Bayley, N., 21[3], *51*

Bèbe, M., *122, 142*
Beintema, D., 22[8], *51, 143*
Benfiedl, G., 266[46], *277*
Berenberg, W., 11[39], *17*
Bice, H., 8[32], *17*
Biehl, R., 45[26], *52*
Bijou, S., 67[44], *71*
Birch, H., [49], *72*
Birdsong, J., 65[32], *71*
Blankenstein, M. V., *122, 142*
Bleck, E., 261[34, 35], *277*
Blook, J., 67[45], *71*
Blodgett, W., 260[19], *276*
Bly, L., 77[3, 4], *121, 142*, 207[6], *256*
Bobath, B., 23[13], *51*, 63[26, 27], *70*, 77[5], *121, 122, 142, 202*, 208[7], *256*, 261[25], *276*

Bobath, K., 22[6], 23[13], *51,*
    63[26, 27], *70,* 77[5], *121,*
    122, 142, 208[7], *256,*
    261[25], *276*
Boland, T., 258[3], *275*
Bosma, F., 57[8], *69*
Bosma, J. F., 57[6], *69, 202*
Bower, T. G. R., *122, 142*
Brazelton, T. B., *122, 142*
Breakey, A., 8[29], *17*
Brissaud, E., 8, *17*
Brown, J., 57[7], *69*
Brown, M., 260[12, 13, 14, 15],
    275
Burgess, D., 8, *16*
Butterfield, E., 55[4], *69*

Camp, B., 41[24], *52*
Caplan, F., *122, 143*
Caplan, T., *122, 143*
Capute, A., 33[20], 45[26], *52,*
    143
Carlsen, P., 265[42], *277*
Carlson, E., 259[8], *275*
Casaer, P., *122, 143*
Cavins, G., 55[4], *69*
Cazauvielh, J., 1[1], *15*
Cheeni, Y., 31[18], *51*
Chesni, I., *142*
Childs, B., 11[41], *17*
Churchill, J., 11[38, 40, 49],
    12[52], *17, 18*
Chyatte, S., 65[32], *71*
Cicenia, E., 260[16], *276*
Clarke, E., 22[11], *51*
Close, J., 261[36], *277*
Cohen, H., [49], *72*
Colby, J., 5[9], *16*
Colton, K., 8[32], *17*
Connor, F., 60[13], *70*
Connors, C., 68[53], *72*

Cook, C., 58[10], *69*
Cooper, I., 66[40], *71*
Cooper, W., 13[57], *18,* 30[16],
    51, 65[36], *71*
Couch, W., 257[2], *275*
Crosland, J., 260[21], 264[21],
    276
Crothers, B., 10, *17,* 61[16], *70*
Cruickshank, W., 13[59], *18*
Csongradi, J., 261[35], *277*

Danhoff, E., 65[35], *71*
Dargassies, S., 23[12], 31[17, 18],
    33[12], *51*
Davidson, S., 66[39], *71*
Davies, P., 11[43], *17*
Davis, L. F., *203*
Deaver, G., 61[18], 62[19], *70,*
    260[12], *275*
Delacato, C., 261[30, 31], 264[30,
    31], *276*
Delpech, M., 1[2], *15*
Denhoff, E., 64[30], *71*
De Rosa, G., 257[2], *275*
Doman, G., 261[30, 31, 32], 264
    [30, 31, 32], *276*
Doman, R., 62[22], *70,* 261[30,
    31], 264[30, 31], *276*
Doty, R. W., *202*
Drillien, C., 11[42], *17,* 23[14], *51*
Dubowitz, V., 46[30], *52*

Eastman, N., 11[44], *17*
Ellenberg, J., 13[65], *19,* 269[50],
    277
Epstein, L., 269[51], *277*
Evans, P., 11[41], *17*

Fabricant, P., *203*
Falconer, M., 66[39], *71*

Fallstrom, K., 259[6], *275*
Fanaroff, A., 13[67], *19*
Farrell, S., 6[14], *16*
Fay, T., 9, *17*, 62[20], *70*
Finnie, N. R., 59[12], *70, 202*
Fisher, E., 206[2], *256*
Fitzhardinge, P., 13[68], *19*
Footh, V., 260[20], 264[20], *276*
Ford, F., 261[34, 35], *277*
Franco, S., 13[64], 14[64], *19*
Frankenberg, W., 41[24], *52*
Freeman, R., [48], *72*
Freud, S., 5[8], *16, 17*

Gallenstein, J., 259[11], *275*
German, J., 13[57], *18*
Gesell, A., 21[1], 48[1], *51, 122, 143*
Gidoni, E. A., *122, 143*, 206[5], *256*, 261[33], *276*
Gilette, H., 62[23], *70*
Gilman, A., 65[37], *71*
Goldenson, R., 68[50], *72*
Goldstein, A., 41[24], *52*
Goodman, A., 65[37], *71*
Goodman, L., 65[37], *71*
Gordon, S., 45[28], *52*
Gould, S., 62[21], *70*
Gowers, W., 2[6], *16*
Graziani, L., 55[3], *69*
Green, A., 67[43], *71*
Green, E., 67[43], *71*
Green, W., 257[1], *275*
Greenspan, L., 8[20], *16*
Guidubaldi, J., 266[46], *277*

Haas, J. H., *122, 142*
Haberfellner, H., *143*
Hagberg, B., 13, 14[63], 15[63], *18*
Hagberg, G., 13, 14[63], 15[63], *18*

Haring, N., 259[5], *275*
Harris, D., 41[25], *52*
Harryman, S., *143*
Hawkins, R., 67[44], *71*
Hayden, A., 259[5], *275*
Haynes, U., 7[18], *16*, 58[11], *69*
Henderson, J., 13[61], *18*
Herman, R., 65[31, 33], *71*
Hoberman, M., 260[16], *276*
Hochleitner, M., *143, 202*, 265[43], *277*
Hogan, G., 39[22], *52*
Hooker, D., 74[1], *121*
Hopkins, T., 8[32], *17*

Illingworth, R. S., 21[4], 32[4], 34[4], 48[4], *51, 122, 143, 202*
Ilson, J., 261[28], 265[28], *276*
Ingram, A., 260[17], *276*
Ingram, T. T. S., 57[5], *69, 143, 202*

Jackson, H. J., 206[1], *256*
Jackson, J., 21[5], *51*
Janniruberto, A., 74[2], *121*
Jantzin, A., 260[22], *276*
Jenkins, W., 21[2], *51*
Johnson, K., 7[17], *16*
Johnson, M., 261[23, 24], 264[24], *276*
Jones, M., 260[18], *276*

Kalman, E., 13[68], *19*
Katz, A., 6[15], *16*
Keats, S., 65[34], *71*
Kemp, F. H., 58[9], *69, 202*
Kiely, J., 15[71, 72, 73], *19*
Kitchen, W., 13[66], *19*
Kline, M., 68[50], *72*

Knott, M., 63[25], *70*
Koeng, E., *143*, 208[8], *256*
Koenigsberger, R., [48], *18*
Kong, E., 264[39], *277*
Koven, L., 261[29], *276*

Lame, E., 13[57], *18*
Lee, J., 65[38], *71*
Leib, S., 266[46], *277*
Lesch, M., 46[29], *52*
Lind, J., *202*
Little, W., 1[3, 4], 2[5], 3[5],
    11[5], *15, 16*
Logan, K., 260[20], 264[20],
    276
Logan, W., 57[6], *69*
Lord, E., 5, *16*
Louick, D., 258[3], *275*

McDermott, L., 257[1], *275*
McDonald, A., 11[45], *18*
McDowell, F., 65[36, 38], *71*
Magnus, R., 206[3], *256*
Martin, J., 269[51], *277*
Masland, R., 11[49], *18*
Matson, D., 13[56], *18*
Mayer, N., 65[31, 33], *71*
Mecomber, S., 65[31, 33], *71*
Merkatz, I., 7[17], 13[67], *16, 19*
Mike, V., 11[47], *18*, 261[28],
    265[28], *276*
Milani-Comparetti, A., 64, *70*,
    74[2], *121, 122, 143*, 206[5],
    256, 261[33], *276*
Miller, A., 260[22], *276*
Miller, D., 269[49], *277*
Milligan, J., 39[22], *52*
Minear, W., 10[37], *17*
Molnar, G., 45[28], *52*
Moran, P., 261[32], 264[32], *276*

Morgese, A., 65[34], *71*
Morris, S. E., *202*
Mueller, H. A., *202*
Murphy, M., 260[22], *276*

Nagler, A., 11[49], *18*
Nellhaus, G., 29[15], *51*
Nelson, K., 13[65], *19*, 269[50],
    277
Nicholson, J., 264[41], *277*
Nieburg, H., 68[50], *72*
Nieburgs, T., 68[50], *72*
Nordlund, T., 65[34], *71*
Nyhan, W., 46[29], *52*

Olegard, R., 11[50], *18*
Oliver, W., 46[29], *52*
Olow, I., 13[63], 14[63],
    15[63], *18*
O'Malley, C., 22[11], *51*
Ong, B., 11[39], *17*
O'Reilly, D., 8[28], *17*
Osler, W., 2[7], 8, *16*
Osternig, L., 259[11], *275*

Paine, R., 10, *17*, 33[19, 21, 23],
    39[23], *52*, 263[38], *277*
Paneth, N., 15[71, 72, 73], *19*
Pascal, G., 21[2], *51*
Peiper, A., [8], *121, 143*
Perlstein, M., 8[21], 10, 11[21],
    12[21], 13[62], 14[21],
    16, 17, 18
Peterson, F., 8, *16*
Peterson, R., 67[44], *71*
Peyser, A., 22[7], *51*
Phelps, W., 5[12], 8[27], 10[34],
    13[60], *16, 17, 18*, 61[17],
    70
Polani, P., 12[51], *18*

Prechtl, H., 22[8], *51*, 55[2], *69, 143*

Quinton, M. B., 77[6, 7], *121, 143,* 208[8], *256*

Raus, G., 13[59], *18*
Rawlings, G., 13[70], *19*
Rembolt, R., 266[44], *277*
Reynolds, E., 13[69], *19*
Rie, C., 8[26], 9[26], *17*
Roberson, D., 65[32], *71*
Robinson, R., 8[31], *17*
Roboz, P., 12[53], *18*
Roizen, N., 6[14], *16*
Rood, M., 63[24], *70*
Rosenberg, L., 8, 9, *17*
Rosenblith, J. F., *143*
Rosenthal, R., 30[16], *51*, 65[36], *71*
Roth, B., 266[44], *277*
Rowe, R., 261[29], *276*
Rubenstein, J., 6[14], *16, 143*

Sabel, K., 11[50], *18*
Sachs, B., 8, *16*
Saint-Anne Dargassies, S., *122, 142, 143, 144*
Sameroff, A. J., *202*
Scherzer, A. L., 11[47], *18*, 30[16], 33[31], 36[31], 40[31], *51, 52*, 60[14], *70*, 261[28], 265[28], *276*
Schoenberg, B., 12[55], *18*
Schweid, E., 67[44], *71*
Semans, S., 261[26], 262[37], *276, 277*
Shaltenbrand, G., 206[4], *256*
Sherrington, C., 22[10], *51*
Sholl, C., 60[14], *70*
Showacre, J., *202*

Siepp, J., 60[13], *70*
Silver, J., 13[58], *18*, 45[27], *52*
Silver, L., 64[29], *70*
Silverstein, L., 67[45, 46], *71*
Skrotzky, K., 259[11], *275*
Spears, C., 68[51], *72*
Spellacy, W., 12[54], *18*
Spetz, E., 260[17], *276*
Spira, R., 259[10], *275*
Spitzer, A., 269[48], *277*
Staub, J., *203*
Stein, Z., 15[71, 72, 73], *19*
Stephenson, C., 260[16], *276*
Stern, F., *122, 144*
Steward, A., 13[69, 70], *19*
Stewart, M., 260[22], *276*
Stoffel, A., 5, *16*
Stroud, C., 66[39], *71*
Susser, M., 15[71, 72, 73], *19*
Sweet, R., 65[38], *71*

Taft, L., [49], *72*
Tajani, E., 74[2], *121*
Thomas, A., 31[18], *51*
Thossem, T., 266[45], *277*
Throop, F., 257[2], *275*
Tizard, J., 11[43], *17*
Tjossem, T. D., 7[19], *16*, 61[15], *70*
Touwen, B., *122, 144*
Tower, G., 261[27], *276*
Tsauffkirchen, E., *256*
Tscharnuter, I., *203*
Turcan, D., 13[70], *19*

Velasco, M., 55[3], *69*
Vernon, M., 8[30], *17*
Victoria, L., 11[50], *18*
Vining, E., 6[14], *16, 143*
Vlach, V., 55[2], *69*
von Bermuth, H., 55[2], *69*

Voss, D., 63[25], *70*

Wainer, G., 259[9], *275*
Walters, E., 67[43], *71*
Weisz, St., *144*
Weitzman, E., 55[3], *69*
Welbergen, U. R., *122, 142*
White, B., *122, 144*
Wilder, C. N., *203*
Williamson, G., 60[13], *70*
Willoughby, M., *203*
Wilson, J. M., *203*

Wingate, K., 261[23], *276*
Withers, E., 260[17], *276*
Wolf, J., 5[13], *16*, 259[7], *275*
Woods, G., 264[40], *277*
Wright, F., 11[46], *18*
Wright, T., 264[41], *277*

Zapella, M., 55[1], *69*
Zar, J., 266[47], *277*
Zausmer, E., 261[27], *276*
Zuck, F., 261[23], *276*

Subject Index

Assessment concepts
  adaptive behavior, 125-126
  automatic postural reactions, 125
  contractures, 138-142
  developmental milestones, 126-
    128
    change of positions in, 127
    head, trunk control, 126-127
    progression, 127
    supported standing, 128
    upper extremity, 127
  holistic approach, 123
  motor response variability, 130
  movement grading, 130-131
  movement sequencing, 131
  postural alignment, 132-134
    plane 1, 133
    plane 2, 134
    plane 3, 134
  postural stability, 135-138
    dissociated movements, 137-138
    equilibrium reactions, 136
    protective extension, 136-137
    proximal, 135
  postural symmetry, 132

[Assessment concepts]
  postural tonus, 128-130
    abnormal, 129, 130
      associated reactions, 129
      fluctuation of tone, 130
      hypertonicity, 129
      hypotonicity, 129-130
      reciprocal innervation, 130
    normal, 128-129
      strength and distribution, 128
      reciprocal innervation, 129
  primitive reflexes, 132
Assessment procedures
  evaluation positions, 148-151
    prone, 149
    quadruped, 149-150
    sitting, 150-151
    standing and walking, 151
    supine, 148-149
    upper extremity, 151
  evaluation report, 151-152
  feeding evaluation
    biting and chewing, 154-156
    cup drinking, 153
    postural assessment, 152

285

[Assessment procedures]
  [feeding evaluation]
    self-feeding, 156
    spoon feeding, 154
    sucking, 153
  initial evaluation, 146–147
  method, 147
  oral examination, 156–159
    breathing patterns, 159
    posture, tone, structure, 157–
      158
  oral examination
    reflexes, 158–159
    sensitivity, 158
  oral and feeding evaluation, 152–
    159
  parent interview, 147

Cerebral palsy
  acquired, 12
    etiology of, 12
    frequency of, 12
  associated handicaps, 8
  congenital, 11
    etiology of, 11
    frequency of, 11
  definition, 8
    history of, 8
  diagnosis, 42–45
  differential diagnosis, 45–47
  etiology, 11–13
  epidemiology, 13–15
    associated handicaps, 15
    current trends, 15
    degree of severity, 14
    factors affecting, 13
    incidence and prevalence, 13
    types and distribution, 14
  genetic, 13
    pathology of, 12

history, 1–8
[Cerebral palsy]
  [history]
    American Academy for Cerebral
      Palsy and Developmental
      Medicine, 8
    classification systems, 9–11
    early intervention treatment, 7
    etiology theories, 2–5
    Freud, influence of, 5
    and John Little, 1–2
    multispecialty approach, 5
    orthopedic surgery, 1, 5
    physical therapy, 5, 60
  motor classification, 8–11

Development, sensorimotor
  abnormal, 75–76
  and reflex behavior, 75
  fetal movements, 74
  general concepts, 74–76
  postural control, 74–75
Developmental evaluation, 24–42
  developmental milestones, 27
  history of delivery, 26
  history of labor, 26
  history of pregnancy, 25
  neurological examination, 31–40
    soft neurological signs, 39
  past medical history, 29
  physical examination, 29–31
  review of systems, 29
  social and emotional factors, 27–
    29
Diagnosis
  early developmental deficit classi-
    fication, 44
Diagnosis differential
  nonprogressive conditions, 45
  progressive disease, 46–47

Emotional impact, 164

Feeding patterns, 119-121
Functional assessment, 58-60
  management evaluation, 59-60

Guidelines for patient assessment,
  270-271
  initial evaluation, 270
  re-evaluation, 270-271
Guidelines for therapy research,
  271-272

Head control
  abnormal, 78-80
  abnormal extensor tone, 79
  abnormal flexor tone, 79
    primitive posture, 78-79
  normal, 77-78
Home management
  baby carrier, 178
  bathing, 181
  biting and chewing, 192-193
  bottle drinking, 190
  car seats, 170
  carrying, 176-178
  in abnormal development, 176-
    178
  in normal development, 176
  cup drinking, 191
  dressing, 181-185
    choice of clothes, 185
    handling principles in, 185
    in abnormal development, 182
    in normal development, 181-
     182
    positions, 182-185
     prone, 184
     side lying, 183
     sitting, 182-183
     supine, 182

[Home management]
  feeding, 186-194
    positioning, 187-189
    procedures, 190-194
  handling, 178-181
  infant walkers, 171
  jaw control, 189-190
  lifting, 181
  mobility, 185-186
    equipment, 186
  oral hygiene, 194
  positioning and seating, 165-171
    independent sitting, 170
    prone board, 172-176
    prone position, 166-167
     equipment for, 167
  self-feeding, 193
    associated reactions, 193-194
  side lying position, 167-168
    equipment for, 168
  sitting position, 168-170
    abnormal development, 168-169
    equipment for, 169-170
    normal development, 168
  spoon feeding, 192
  standing tables, 171
  standing with support, 171-176
    abnormal, 171
    equipment for, 171-176
    normal, 171
    positioning in, 171
  strollers, 170
  sucking, 190
  supine board, 172-176
Supine position
  abnormal, 166
  equipment for, 166
  normal, 165

Laboratory evaluation, 41-42
Locomotion patterns
  abnormal, 108-111

[Locomotion patterns]
  [abnormal]
    asymmetry in, 110
    commando crawling, 109
    proximal instability in, 110
  normal, 106-107
    amphibian reaction, 106

Motor signs, late emergence, 24

Neurological development, 21-23
  abnormal, 22-23; 53-58
    discordant maturation, 53-54
    oral development deficits, 57-58
    sensory deficits and function,
      55-56
    influence of abnormal tone, 54-
      55
  normal, 21-22

Parent counseling, 164
Posture control, prone
  abnormal, 81-84
  normal, 80-81
Posture control, supine
  abnormal, 86-88
  normal, 84-86
Prescription, 68-69
  for evaluation, 68
  for therapy, 69

Reflex behavior
  abnormal, 56-57
    functional deprivation, 56-57
  assessment concepts, 132
  description, 33-39
  postural reflexes, 33
  primitive reflexes, 33
Research, 266-270
  current status, 266-267

[Research]
  obstacles, 267-270
    environmental influences, 268
    recording and interpreting data,
      269
    sampling bias, 268
    selecting and using test instru-
      ments, 269
    therapist bias, 267-268
    use of controls, 269-270

Sitting
  abnormal, 98-105
    asymmetry, 103
    compensatory flexion in, 100
    excessive extension and, 98
  normal, 93-97
Standing patterns
  abnormal, 116-119
    hypotonicity, 118-119
    positive supporting reaction in,
      117
  normal, 112-115
    reflex walking, 113

Testing, psychological, 40-41
Therapy methods, 60-64
  Bobath and N.D.T., 63-64
  Crothers, 61
  Deaver, 61
  Fay-Doman, 62
  Kabat-Knott, 63
  Phelps, 61
  Rood, 63
Therapy studies, 263-266
  control studies, 265-266
  narrative case reviews, 263-264
  with specific instruments, 264-
    265

Treatment
neurodevelopmental approach,
206-208
Treatment assessment, 257-263
concepts, 257-259
procedures, 259-263
activities of daily living, 260
case histories, 259
clinical assessments, 262-263
development profiles, 261
functional inventories, 260
motor ability tests, 261
narrative reports, 259
pattern analysis, 261
skill tests, 260
Treatment modalities
behavior modification, 67
controversial treatments, 68
medication, 64-65
orthotic devices and equipment,
65-66
special education, 67-68
social and mental health services,
67
surgery, 66-67
therapy methods, 60-64
Treatment principles, 208-211
components of movement, 209
grading of stimulation, 208-209
handling, 210-211
dynamic versus static, 209
Treatment procedures, 211-253
body righting on head, 218-219
facilitation of walking, 248-253
four point crawling, 240-242
head control, 212-215
lateral head righting, 215

[Treatment procedures]
neck elongation, 216-217
protective extension of arms,
236-240
protective extension of arms
and shoulder girdle stability,
237-240
rolling and crawling, 225-230
amphibian reaction in, 225-228
rotation within body axis, 228-
230
standing balance, 247-248
standing and walking, 242-253
foot balance, 245
foot-eye coordination, 243
foot position, 243-244
weight bearing in flexion, 245-
247
trunk control, 220-225
prone flexion-extension, 220
righting reactions in sitting,
221-247
supine flexion-extension, 221
upper extremity weight bearing,
230-235
dissociation movements in,
231-233
and pelvic control, 230-231
and reclined sitting, 234-235

Weight bearing, upper
abnormal, 91-93
and associated movements, 91
scapular protraction and, 91
normal, 88-91
shoulder stability in, 89